KV-508-797

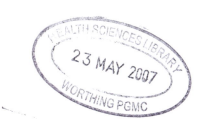

HEALTH SCIENCES LIBRARY
23 MAY 2007
WORTHING PGMC

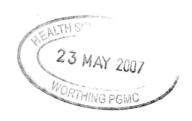

HEALTH S
23 MAY 2007
WORTHING PGMC

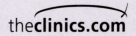

MAGNETIC RESONANCE IMAGING CLINICS

OF NORTH AMERICA

MR Imaging of the Female Pelvis

Guest Editor

MICHÈLE A. BROWN, MD

November 2006 • Volume 14 • Number 4

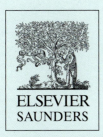

ELSEVIER
SAUNDERS

An imprint of Elsevier, Inc
PHILADELPHIA LONDON TORONTO MONTREAL SYDNEY TOKYO

W.B. SAUNDERS COMPANY
A Divison of Elsevier Inc.

Elsevier Inc. ● 1600 John F. Kennedy Boulevard ● Suite 1800 ●
Philadelphia, Pennsylvania 19103-2899

http://www.mri.theclinics.com

MRI CLINICS OF NORTH AMERICA Volume 14, Number 4
November 2006 ISSN 1064-9689, ISBN 13: 978-1-4160-4332-4, ISBN 10: 1-4160-4332-2

Editor: Lisa Richman

Copyright © 2007 by Elsevier Inc. All rights reserved. No part of this publication may be
reproduced or transmitted in any form or by any means, electronic or mechanical, including
photocopy, recording, or any information retrieval system, without permission from the
Publisher.

Single photocopies of single articles may be made for personal use as allowed by national
copyright laws. Permission of the publisher and payment of a fee is required for all other
photocopying, including multiple or systematic copying, copying for advertising or promotional
purposes, resale, and all forms of document delivery. Special rates are available for educational
institutions that wish to make photocopies for non-profit educational classroom use. Permissions
may be sought directly from Elsevier's Rights Department in Philadelphia, PA, USA: phone: (+1)
215 239 3804, fax: (+1) 215 239 3805, e-mail: healthpermissions@elsevier.com. Requests also
may be completed on-line via the Elsevier homepage (http://www.elsevier.com/locate/
permissions). In the USA, users may clear permissions and make payments through the
Copyright Clearance Center, Inc., 222 Rosewood Drive, "Danvers, MA 01923, USA; phone: (978)
750-8400, fax: (978) 750-4744, and in the UK through the Copyright Licensing Agency Rapid
Clearance Service (CLARCS), 90 Tottenham Court Road, London W1P 0LP, UK; phone: (+44)
171 436 5931; fax: (+44) 171 436 3986. Other countries may have a local reprographic rights
agency for payments.

Reprints:.For copies of 100 or more, of articles in this publication, please contact the Commercial
Reprints Department, Elsevier Inc., 360 Park Avenue South, New York, New York 10010-1710. Tel.
(212) 633-3813, Fax: (212) 462-1935, email: reprints@elsevier.com.

The ideas and opinions expressed in *Magnetic Resonance Imaging Clinics of North America* do not
necessarily reflect those of the Publisher. The Publisher does not assume any responsibility for
any injury and/or damage to persons or property arising out of or related to any use of the
material contained in this periodical. The reader is advised to check the appropriate medical
literature and the product information currently provided by the manufacturer of each drug to be
administered to verify the dosage, the method and duration of administration, or
contraindications. It is the responsibility of the treating physician or other health care
professional, relying on independent experience and knowledge of the patient, to determine drug
dosages and the best treatment for the patient. Mention of any product in this issue should not be
construed as endorsement by the contributors, editors, or the Publisher of the product or
manufacturers' claims.

Magnetic Resonance Imaging Clinics of North America (ISSN 1064-9689) is published quarterly by
Elsevier Inc., 360 Park Avenue South, New York, NY 10010-1710. Months of issue are February,
May, August, and November. Business and Editorial Offices: 1600 John F. Kennedy Blvd., Suite
1800, Philadelphia, PA 19103-2899. Customer Service Office: 6277 Sea Harbor Drive, Orlando,
FL 32887-4800. Periodicals postage paid at New York, NY and additional mailing offices.
Subscription prices are $226.00 per year (US individuals), $336.00 per year (US institutions),
$110.00 per year (US students), $253.00 per year (Canadian individuals), $413.00 per year
(Canadian institutions), $149.00 per year (Canadian students), $308.00 per year (international
individuals), $413.00 per year (international institutions), and $149.00 per year (international
students). International air speed delivery is included in all *Clinics* subscription prices. All prices
are subject to change without notice. **POSTMASTER:** Send address changes to *Magnetic
Resonance Imaging Clinics,* Elsevier Periodicals Customer Service, 6277 Sea Harbor Drive,
Orlando, FL 32887-4800. **Customer Service: 1-800-654-2452 (US). From outside of the US,
call 1-407-345-4000.**

Magnetic Resonance Imaging Clinics of North America is covered in the *RSNA Index of Imaging
Literature, Index Medicus, MEDLINE,* and *EMBASE/Excerpta Medica.*

Printed in the United States of America.

MR IMAGING OF THE FEMALE PELVIS

GUEST EDITOR

MICHÈLE A. BROWN, MD
Assistant Professor, Department of Radiology,
University of California, San Diego Medical Center,
San Diego, California

CONTRIBUTORS

MICHÈLE A. BROWN, MD
Assistant Professor, Department of Radiology,
University of California, San Diego Medical Center,
San Diego, California

INBAL COHEN, MD
Neuroradiology Fellow, Department of Radiology,
University of California, San Diego Medical Center,
University of California, San Diego, San Diego,
California

HENRIQUE R. DE ABREU, MD
Clinical Research Fellow, Department of Radiology,
University of California, San Diego Medical Center,
San Diego, California

ROSALIND B. DIETRICH, MD
Professor of Radiology and Director of MRI,
Department of Radiology, University of California,
San Diego Medical Center, University of California,
San Diego, San Diego, California

NIALL T.M. GALLOWAY, MD
Director, Emory Continence Center, and Associate
Professor, Department of Urology, Emory
University School of Medicine, Atlanta, Georgia

CLAUDIA P. HUERTAS, MD
Clinical Research Fellow, Department of Radiology,
University of North Carolina, Chapel Hill, North
Carolina; Section Body MRI, Department of
Radiology, Instituto Neurologico de Antioquia,
Medellin, Colombia

SHAHID M. HUSSAIN, MD, PhD
Herbert B. Saichek Professor of Radiology,
and Director of Body MR Imaging, and Chief,
Abdominal Imaging, Department of Radiology,
University of Nebraska Medical Center, Omaha,
Nebraska

DIEGO R. MARTIN, MD, PhD
Director of Body MR Imaging, and Professor
of Radiology, Department of Radiology, Emory
University School of Medicine, Emory University
Hospital, Atlanta, Georgia

JENNIFER M. OLIVETO, MD
Assistant Professor, Department of Radiology,
University of Nebraska Medical Center, Omaha,
Nebraska

AYTEKIN OTO, MD
Associate Professor of Radiology, and Vice
Chairman for Research Affairs, and Director
of Body Imaging, Department of Radiology,
University of Texas Medical Branch at Galveston,
Galveston, Texas

KHALIL SALMAN, MD
Department of Radiology, Emory University School
of Medicine, Atlanta, Georgia

RICHARD C. SEMELKA, MD
Professor, Department of Radiology, University
of North Carolina, Chapel Hill, North Carolina

INDRA C. VAN DEN BOS, MD
Department of Radiology, Erasmus Medical Center,
Rotterdam, The Netherlands

CHESTER C. WILMOT, MD
Instructor, Department of Urology, Emory
University School of Medicine, Atlanta, Georgia

MR IMAGING OF THE FEMALE PELVIS

Volume 14 • Number 4 • November 2006

Contents

technique and the imaging characteristics of malignant disease of the uterine corpus and cervix.

MR Imaging Evaluation of the Adnexa   471

Claudia P. Huertas, Michèle A. Brown, and Richard C. Semelka

MR imaging has become an important tool in the evaluation of patients with adnexal disease, and its role continues to evolve. Some benign entities can be diagnosed by MR imaging with a high grade of confidence, such as teratomas, endometriomas, simple and hemorrhagic cysts, fibromas, and hydrosalpinx. In cases of malignant lesions, MR imaging may be more accurate than other modalities for lesion characterization, staging, and follow-up.

MR Imaging Evaluation of Acute Abdominal Pain During Pregnancy   489

Aytekin Oto

MR imaging enables diagnosis of a variety of maternal diseases presenting as acute abdominal pain in pregnant patients. MR imaging is a valuable complement to ultrasound in the determination of the exact etiology of acute abdominal pain, and it is important for the radiologist to recognize the MR imaging appearance of common causes of acute abdominal pain during pregnancy. This article reviews the MR imaging technique and findings of various abnormalities causing acute abdominal pain in pregnant patients.

Fetal MR Imaging   503

Rosalind B. Dietrich and Inbal Cohen

Ultrasonography is the primary prenatal screening modality used in the evaluation of the fetus and the maternal pelvis. However, fetal MR imaging plays a complementary role to prenatal ultrasound in the evaluation of the fetus with suspected abnormalities. MR imaging's role includes confirming or excluding possible lesions, defining their full extent, aiding in their characterization, and demonstrating other associated abnormalities. As newer techniques such as diffusion imaging, MR spectroscopy, and functional studies are used more widely, it is hoped that additional information will be made available by this modality to physicians evaluating and taking care of fetuses.

MR Imaging Evaluation of the Pelvic Floor for the Assessment of Vaginal Prolapse and Urinary Incontinence   523

Diego R. Martin, Khalil Salman, Chester C. Wilmot, and Niall T.M. Galloway

Pelvic MR imaging using the combination of motion-insensitive T2-weighted single-shot fast spin echo and high soft tissue resolution standard T2-weighted fast spin echo techniques has helped to identify soft tissue abnormalities that directly correlate with the clinical and intraoperative findings related to pelvic floor prolapse. In particular, the authors have shown that pelvic MR imaging has the ability to identify changes related to uterosacral ligament disruption and to document the corrective changes after surgical repair of this ligament. In the future, pelvic MR imaging is expected to play a progressively larger role in preoperative planning for complex or uncertain cases and for more detailed evaluation of repair in cases that do not show good symptomatic response. Pelvic MR imaging should also help to document and advance knowledge of surgical repair methodology.

MR Imaging of the Female Pelvis at 3T 537

Shahid M. Hussain, Indra C. van den Bos, Jennifer M. Oliveto, and Diego R. Martin

The recent development of the transmit-receive body coil and the dedicated torso phased-array radio frequency receive coil for 3.0T MR imaging systems has promoted a move toward higher-field, whole-body MR imaging, including pelvic MR imaging. The female pelvis is an anatomic area that may benefit particularly from the advantages of high-field systems. In this article, the authors present their initial experience with the optimization of sequences for MR imaging of the female pelvis at 3.0T, and include a short description of parallel imaging. They compare some of the physical properties of 1.5T and 3.0T, discuss some of the challenges during sequence optimization for the female pelvis at 3.0T, and give examples of female pelvic abnormalities.

Index 545

THE CLINICS ARE NOW AVAILABLE ONLINE!

Access your subscription at:
www.theclinics.com

GOAL STATEMENT

The goal of *Magnetic Resonance Imaging Clinics of North America* is to keep practicing physicians up to date with current clinical practice by providing timely articles reviewing the state of the art in patient care.

ACCREDITATION

The *Magnetic Resonance Imaging Clinics of North America* is planned and implemented in accordance with the Essential Areas and Policies of the Accreditation Council for Continuing Medical Education (ACCME) through the joint sponsorship of the University of Virginia School of Medicine and Elsevier. The University of Virginia School of Medicine is accredited by the ACCME to provide continuing medical education for physicians.

The University of Virginia School of Medicine designates this educational activity for a maximum of 15 *AMA PRA Category 1 Credits*™. Physicians should only claim credit commensurate with the extent of their participation in the activity.

The American Medical Association has determined that physicians not licensed in the US who participate in this CME activity are eligible for 15 *AMA PRA Category 1 Credits*™.

Credit can be earned by reading the text material, taking the CME examination online at http://www.theclinics.com/home/cme, and completing the evaluation. After taking the test, you will be required to review any and all incorrect answers. Following completion of the test and evaluation, your credit will be awarded and you may print your certificate.

FACULTY DISCLOSURE/CONFLICT OF INTEREST

The University of Virginia School of Medicine, as an ACCME accredited provider, endorses and strives to comply with the Accreditation Council for Continuing Medical Education (ACCME) Standards of Commercial Support, Commonwealth of Virginia statutes, University of Virginia policies and procedures, and associated federal and private regulations and guidelines on the need for disclosure and monitoring of proprietary and financial interests that may affect the scientific integrity and balance of content delivered in continuing medical education activities under our auspices.

The University of Virginia School of Medicine requires that all CME activities accredited through this institution be developed independently and be scientifically rigorous, balanced and objective in the presentation/discussion of its content, theories and practices.

All authors/editors participating in an accredited CME activity are expected to disclose to the readers relevant financial relationships with commercial entities occurring within the past 12 months (such as grants or research support, employee, consultant, stock holder, member of speakers bureau, etc.). The University of Virginia School of Medicine will employ appropriate mechanisms to resolve potential conflicts of interest to maintain the standards of fair and balanced education to the reader. Questions about specific strategies can be directed to the Office of Continuing Medical Education, University of Virginia School of Medicine, Charlottesville, Virginia.

The authors/editors listed below have identified no professional or financial affiliations for themselves or their spouse/partner:

Michelle A. Brown, MD (Guest Editor); Inbal Cohen, MD; Henrique R. de Abreu, MD; Rosalind B. Dietrich, MD; Niall T.M. Galloway, MD; Claudia P. Huertas, MD; Shahid M. Hussain, MD, PhD; Diego R. Martin, MD, PhD; Jennifer M. Oliveto, MD; Aytekin Oto, MD; Lisa Richman (Acquisitions Editor); Khalil Salman, MD; Indra C. van den Bos, MD; and, Chester C. Wilmot, MD.

The authors/editors listed below identified the following professional or financial affiliations for themselves or their spouse/partner:

Richard C. Semelka, MD serves on the Speaker's Bureau for BRACCO.

Disclosure of Discussion of non-FDA approved uses for pharmaceutical products and/or medical devices:

The University of Virginia School of Medicine, as an ACCME provider, requires that all faculty presenters identify and disclose any "off label" uses for pharmaceutical and medical device products. The University of Virginia School of Medicine recommends that each physician fully review all the available data on new products or procedures prior to instituting them with patients.

TO ENROLL

To enroll in the Magnetic Resonance Imaging Clinics of North America Continuing Medical Education program, call customer service at 1-800-654-2452 or visit us online at www.theclinics.com/home/cme. The CME program is available to subscribers for an additional fee of $99.95.

MAGNETIC
RESONANCE
IMAGING CLINICS

Magn Reson Imaging Clin N Am 14 (2007) xi

Preface

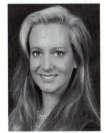

Michèle A. Brown, MD
Guest Editor

Michèle A. Brown, MD
Department of Radiology
University of California
San Diego Medical Center
200 West Arbor Drive
San Diego, CA 92103-8756, USA

E-mail address:
m9brown@ucsd.edu

MR imaging plays an increasing large role in the diagnosis and management of gynecologic conditions. It is certain that MR provides in vivo imaging of the female pelvis with a resolution and tissue contrast impossible to achieve by any other modality, and this has led in many cases to new understanding of anatomy and physiology. Despite its obvious advantages for evaluation of female pelvic disease, MR imaging remains a surprisingly underutilized tool in many centers.

In this issue, current MR techniques are described, and imaging appearances of benign and malignant gynecologic conditions are reviewed. Many common uterine and adnexal disease processes are illustrated along with less common disorders that are well demonstrated by MR imaging, such as those encountered during pregnancy and the postpartum period. A unique diagnostic challenge is the pregnant patient who has acute abdominal pain, and the use of MR imaging in these patients is reviewed in a separate article in this issue. In recent years, fast imaging techniques have expanded the role of female pelvic MR to include evaluation of the pelvic floor and fetus. Novel work using MR imaging to assess urinary incontinence and uterine prolapse is described in this issue, and a thorough review of fetal MR imaging is provided with emphasis on fetal neuroimaging. As the industry moves toward higher-field imaging, there is a need to explore the advantages and challenges associated with adapting female pelvic protocols to 3T systems. The final article of this issue addresses optimization strategies for currently available 3T scanners and equipment, and outlines technical improvements that will facilitate successful high-field MR imaging of the female pelvis in the future.

1064-9689/07/$ – see front matter © 2007 Elsevier Inc. All rights reserved.
doi:10.1016/j.mric.2007.02.003

ELSEVIER
SAUNDERS

MAGNETIC
RESONANCE
IMAGING CLINICS

Magn Reson Imaging Clin N Am 14 (2007) 431–437

Future Directions in MR Imaging of the Female Pelvis

Michèle A. Brown, MD[a],*, Diego R. Martin, MD, PhD[b],
Richard C. Semelka, MD[c]

- ■ High-field MR imaging
- ■ Parallel imaging
- ■ Contrast agents
- ■ Diffusion-weighted imaging and MR spectroscopy
- ■ MR-guided intervention
- ■ Summary
- ■ References

MR imaging plays an increasingly large role in the diagnosis and management of gynecologic conditions. Clinical research using currently available techniques has expanded the application of MR imaging over the past 2 decades. With the ongoing development of new technology, the role of MR imaging is likely to expand even further.

The movement toward higher-field systems requires adaptation of techniques for female pelvis imaging, to achieve acceptable image quality, a goal that is facilitated by parallel imaging methods. In addition to higher-field strengths, female pelvic MR imaging soon may employ contrast agents other than those based on gadolinium, and may include techniques such as diffusion-weighted imaging and MR spectroscopy. Also, the scope of female pelvic MR now extends beyond diagnostic imaging; it is used increasingly to guide intervention to treat gynecologic disease. This article focuses on these select areas of development, which are likely to have an immediate or future impact on MR imaging of the female pelvis.

High-field MR imaging

A technical review of the relative benefits of, and challenges for, abdominal-pelvic imaging at 3 T, in contrast to 1.5 T, has been discussed previously [1], and is reviewed further in an article by Hussain and colleagues elsewhere in this issue. The essential advantage of high-field MR imaging is an increase in signal-to-noise ratio (SNR), which depends on the main magnetic field strength, B_0. Thus, SNR is increased twofold using a 3 T system, compared with a 1.5 T system.

The challenge of imaging at 3 T is to be able to convert sequences, previously optimized for a balance between speed and contrast on the 1.5 T system, while fully capitalizing on the potential increased SNR. Major limitations encountered when imaging at 3 T include (1) increased specific absorption rates (SAR) that then require adoption of modifications for most breath-hold rapid acquisition sequences; (2) increased problems of signal inhomogeneities that arise from the greater shimming

[a] Department of Radiology, University of California, San Diego Medical Center, 200 West Arbor Drive, San Diego, CA 92103-8756, USA
[b] Department of Radiology, Emory University School of Medicine, Emory University Hospital, Building A, AT622, 1365 Clifton Road NE, Atlanta, GA 30322, USA
[c] Department of Radiology, University of North Carolina, 101 Manning Drive CB#7510, Chapel Hill, NC 27599-7510, USA
* Corresponding author.
E-mail address: m9brown@ucsd.edu (M.A. Brown).

1064-9689/07/$ – see front matter © 2007 Elsevier Inc. All rights reserved.
mri.theclinics.com

doi:10.1016/j.mric.2007.01.005

challenge for the extrinsic magnetic field; (3) intrinsic field distortions due to increased susceptibility effects and chemical shift effects; and (4) signal shading problems magnified by dielectric effects increased at higher field strengths (Fig. 1).

Although certain sequences require compromises for implementation at T, including single-shot T2 and balanced-echo techniques [1], the authors have found that certain other sequence techniques benefit from imaging at the higher field strength. These include the 3-D gradient-echo and fast spin-echo (FSE), including turbo variants of this technique.

Standard FSE is not limited by SAR effects, because of the relatively long repetition time (TR) and short echo-train lengths, and can take advantage more fully of the increased SNR at T. For example, the authors have been able to employ FSE for high-resolution imaging in the pelvis approaching 800 phase lines of resolution in approximately 4 minutes of scanning time (Fig. 2).

Three-dimensional gradient echo (GRE) may be implemented optimally at 3 T by taking advantage of the higher signal, to increase the bandwidth, thus allowing a decrease in the echo time (TE) and TR. The benefits include a reduction in susceptibility effects from the shorter TE, and a reduction in scanning time by lowering the TR. The time saving may be converted into higher resolution images. The authors acquire images routinely with less than 2 mm isotropic voxels within a breath hold. This degree of spatial resolution has the added benefit of facilitating multiplanar postprocessing reconstructions.

Because of the current advantages and disadvantages of 3 T imaging, consideration should be made before imaging a particular patient at 3 T rather than 1.5 T. For instance, it has been suggested that fetal imaging not be performed at 3 T because of prominent standing wave effects from amniotic fluid, as well as concerns regarding safety [2]. However, with careful optimization of imaging parameters, it has been shown that high-quality images can be obtained at 3 T with short scan times and acceptable SAR in patients who have various gynecologic diseases [3].

Although excellent quality images of the pelvis are obtainable on the 3 T system, with potentially improved image quality for certain sequence techniques, it remains to be demonstrated that diagnostic improvements are associated with these differences.

Parallel imaging

Parallel imaging acquires data from an array of radiofrequency coils over a specified volume. The sensitivity profiles of the individual elements are calibrated and the gradient phase-encoding steps are reduced, resulting in decreased imaging times or increased resolution within the same amount of time.

Parallel imaging techniques may be divided into two main classes [4]. One class calculates missing lines in k-space before Fourier transformation, whereas the other acts after Fourier transformation, reconstructing a reduced field of view (FOV) image for each coil element before joining (and "unwrapping") the images to form a complete FOV image without aliasing. The first class consists of the k-spaced based techniques, such as simultaneous acquisition of spatial harmonics (SMASH) [5] and generalized autocalibrating partially parallel acquisition (GRAPPA) [6]. GRAPPA differs from SMASH in that no separate calibration acquisition is needed, some improvement in SNR is achieved, and certain specific artifacts are improved. The second class consists of the image-based methods, such as sensitivity encoding (SENSE) [7], array

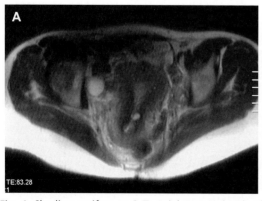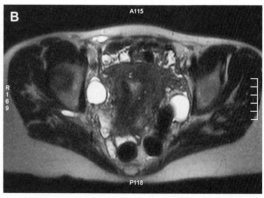

Fig. 1. Shading artifact at 3 T. Axial T2-weighted echo-train spin-echo (ETSE) images of the same patient obtained at 3 T (*A*) and 1.5 T (*B*) show nonuniform signal with a large area of signal loss on the 3 T image (*A*), not seen at 1.5 T (*B*).

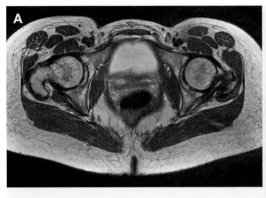

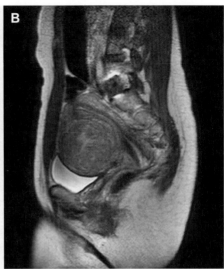

Fig. 2. Example of 3 T MR imaging of the pelvis, showing the capacity to obtain high-resolution and high-contrast T2-weighted ETSE and good contrast single-shot breath-hold images. The axial ETSE image (*A*) was obtained with a resolution of 775 phase lines, 36 cm × 36 cm field of view, TR of 2400 ms, TE of 70 ms, and with an acquisition time of 4 minutes. This image demonstrates the capacity to obtain approximately twice the resolution without an increase in the acquisition time, as compared with 1.5 T. Excellent contrast is achieved and the signal is relatively uniform, without noticeable problems with shading (see text). The sagittal T2-weighted single-shot technique (*B*) was acquired through the midline pelvis, and shows a large anterior uterine fibroid pushing on the endometrium. The contrast in this image is of good quality. The signal homogeneity in the cranio-caudad direction is uniform, despite the large field imaged in the sagittal plane.

spatial sensitivity encoding technique (ASSET), and the autocalibrating modified SENSE (mSENSE). Each method has advantages and disadvantages, depending on the primary goals of imaging. For instance, nonautocalibrating methods such as SENSE may be better if speed is most important, whereas GRAPPA has the advantage of providing smaller FOV images without debilitating artifact [8]. Although currently limited to a specific vendor, the choice of methods likely will become larger as more parallel imaging products are made available commercially.

Common clinical applications of parallel imaging, based on its ability to decrease acquisition time, include cardiac imaging, angiography, enterography, and dynamic imaging of the liver and kidneys. Regarding female pelvic imaging, many advantages are seen at high-field strengths; parallel imaging addresses problems such as increased T2* effects in long echo-train sequences, increased SAR, and increased acoustic noise that occurs as a result of rapid gradient switching [9]. Unique artifacts may occur, such as calibration-related ghosts, increased noise in regions of relatively low signal, and aliasing artifacts in the phase-encoding direction if the prescribed FOV is not large enough (Fig. 3). Such artifacts are minimized by proper technique. As described in a review by Glockner and colleagues [8], parallel imaging has several additional potential applications. For example, the technique may be used to increase SNR, obtain reduced FOV images without wrap, and reduce motion artifacts by allowing adjustments in parameters not possible without parallel imaging. As

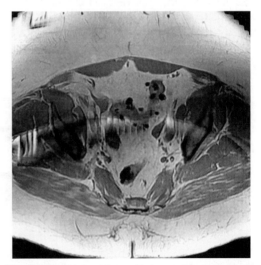

Fig. 3. Parallel imaging: aliasing artifact. Axial T1-weighted gradient-echo image obtained using ASSET with an acceleration factor of two. In the center of the image is a debilitating artifact. This type of artifact can be reduced by increasing the FOV.

experience and availability grow, parallel imaging will probably be used in new ways as a highly versatile tool for image optimization.

Contrast agents

Extracellular gadolinium chelates are the contrast agents used most commonly in MR imaging. New and developing MR contrast agents with potential applications in the female pelvis include gadolinium-based blood pool agents, iron-based agents, and numerous antibody- and peptide-based agents under investigation for molecular imaging. Of these, perhaps the most immediately applicable to gynecologic disease are the iron oxide agents, which show promise for lymph node imaging. Iron oxide particles have been used for various applications in clinical imaging. Unlike the gadolinium-based contrast molecules, iron-based agents are coated crystals, which have an array of sizes. Tissue-specificity depends in large part on particle size. Particles of approximately 200 nm diameter (eg, ferumoxide) are removed quickly from the bloodstream by the reticuloendothelial system and accumulate mostly within Kupffer cells in the liver, whereas ultrasmall particles (<50 nm diameter) remain in the blood pool for a longer period of time [10]. Such ultrasmall superparamagnetic iron oxide (USPIO) particles can be used as tissue-specific agents to image spleen, bone marrow, and lymph nodes. Because the concentration of USPIO in lymph nodes harboring tumor is reduced, malignant lymph nodes remain relatively hyperintense, compared with benign lymph nodes. Improved accuracy of MR imaging for lymph node staging has been reported in pelvic malignancies, including endometrial and cervical cancer [11,12]. In a recent study using a rabbit model, USPIO-enhanced MR imaging was more accurate than positron emission tomography-CT for the detection of malignant pelvic lymph nodes [13]. Because lymph node imaging requires high-resolution sequences with long imaging times, the technique is well-suited for evaluation of tumors of the head and neck or pelvis, and less well suited for tumors involving the upper abdomen.

USPIOs provide targeted imaging of macrophages in lymph nodes; numerous other agents under investigation provide targeted imaging on the molecular level using agents such as labeled antibodies or peptides. Important modalities used for molecular imaging include radionuclide techniques, optics, and MR. MR imaging carries certain advantages, such as higher spatial resolution and the capability of providing simultaneous anatomic and physiologic information. In discussions of molecular imaging contrast media, individual agents or molecular probes are often divided into three general categories. Such probes may be nonspecific, targeted, or activatable "smart" probes, which are detectable only after interaction with a specific target in vivo [14]. Most contrast media in current use are of the nonspecific type, which includes extracellular gadolinium agents. Targeted and activatable agents are more specific and may detect, for example, surface receptors or enzymes.

Numerous targeted and smart agents have been developed for MR imaging, or gadolinium or iron oxide particles associated with proteins or monoclonal antibodies, to image various diseases, including tumor, inflammation, and apoptosis. Smart agents include those activated by enzyme designs and magnetic nanoparticles that can be used to detect molecular interactions by MR imaging. Such magnetic nanosensors have been used to detect DNA, proteins, viruses, and enzymatic activity [15].

Diffusion-weighted imaging and MR spectroscopy

Diffusion-weighted imaging is based on quantification of the molecular motion of water. Similar to T1 and T2, the apparent diffusion coefficient is a tissue property that can be used to help distinguish between normal and abnormal tissue. Abdominal and pelvic applications of diffusion-weighted imaging have been limited by normal physiologic motion, caused by breathing, peristalsis, and vascular

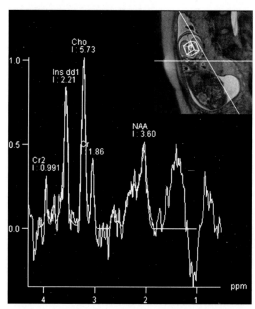

Fig. 4. Fetal brain spectroscopy. Single voxel spectroscopy of the fetal brain using a point-resolved spectroscopy sequence with a TE of 30 ms and a voxel size of 2 × 2 × 2 cm. (*Courtesy of* Rosalind Dietrich, MD, San Diego, CA.)

flow, that overpowers the relatively small-amplitude motion of diffusion. Using ultrafast sequences that essentially are devoid of physiologic motion, it is possible to evaluate structures in the abdomen and pelvis. The technique has been applied successfully to the study of the liver, pancreas, and kidneys [16]. Naganawa and colleagues [17] found that the apparent diffusion coefficient of a cervix with cancer differed significantly from that of a normal cervix and changed after treatment with radiation or chemotherapy, suggesting a possible role in detection and surveillance of cervical cancer. Diffusion-weighted imaging can be accomplished in the fetal brain as well [18,19], for which important applications potentially include early identification of hypoxic-ischemic change.

MR spectroscopy is a means of examining metabolism. Resonances of various metabolites are identified, based on local changes in resonant frequency due to different chemical environments. As with diffusion-weighted imaging, MR spectroscopy has been used mostly in brain imaging, but its use in abdominopelvic imaging is growing. Currently, the most common application of MR spectroscopy within the abdomen and pelvis involves prostate cancer, for which MR spectroscopy has been shown to improve accuracy based on differences in metabolite ratios in cancerous versus benign tissue [20]. More recently, applications have been investigated in the breast, heart, liver, pancreas, kidneys, and cervix [21–26]. Mahon and colleagues [26] found that MR spectroscopy obtained using an endovaginal coil produced characteristic spectra of invasive cervical cancer that could be differentiated from spectra obtained in normal patients. MR spectroscopy can also be performed in the fetal brain, where it may provide additional prognostic information in cases of subtle morphologic abnormalities (Fig. 4) [27].

MR-guided intervention

Interventional MR imaging involves dynamic MR guidance for biopsies, neurosurgery, and various minimally invasive and percutaneous therapies. Tissue biopsies have been performed using MR guidance in nearly every organ system, and therapeutic techniques such as radiotherapy, thermal

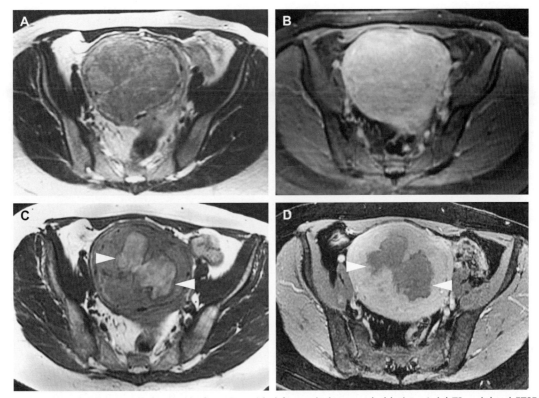

Fig. 5. Uterine leiomyoma, before and after MR-guided focused ultrasound ablation. Axial T2-weighted ETSE (*A, C*) and post-gadolinium, fat-suppressed, T1-weighted (*B, D*) images obtained before (*A, B*) and after (*C, D*) MR-guided focused ultrasound ablation of leiomyoma. A large uterine leiomyoma is seen (*A*) with homogeneous enhancement (*B*) before ablation. After the procedure, an irregular region of infarction is seen centrally within the mass (*arrowheads; C, D*).

ablation, cryoablation, laser therapy, and microwave therapy have been applied with MR guidance to a number of sites, including the brain, breast, heart, prostate, bone, uterus, and blood vessels [28].

One therapeutic method being developed with applications in the female pelvis is focused ultrasound surgery (FUS). FUS uses acoustic energy to heat a limited volume of tissue at a prescribed location within the body. Clinical trials are currently underway for the treatment of uterine leiomyomas. MR is used for imaging guidance, tumor definition, and measurement of effective thermal dose. Unlike thermal ablation techniques using probes, the treated area of FUS is small and the thermal gradient is narrow, leading to more complete necrosis and sparing of surrounding tissue [29]. Typically, imaging follow-up is performed with contrast-enhanced MR imaging, with treated tumors showing areas of nonenhancement and a variable decrease in size from pretreatment images (Fig. 5). It has been reported that diffusion-weighted imaging can be used to monitor therapy, potentially eliminating the need for contrast injection [30].

Although limited data are available regarding clinical outcome, one study reported that 51% of 82 patients reached target symptom reduction at 12 months after MR-guided FUS of symptomatic uterine leiomyomas [31]. FUS was found to have an excellent safety profile, and patients returned to work an average of 1 day after the procedure, compared with the 13 days previously reported for patients undergoing uterine artery embolization, and 6 weeks for those undergoing transabdominal myomectomy or hysterectomy. More clinical trials are needed; however, MR-guided FUS appears to be a promising alternative for treatment of symptomatic leiomyomas.

Summary

Ongoing advances in technology will continue to affect the practice of MR imaging. High-field imaging may become a standard of care, and its success will be aided greatly by parallel imaging techniques. Contrast media remains a focus of active development, with more approved agents becoming available in the near future. In the more distant future, molecular imaging could revolutionize not only MR imaging but also medical imaging as a whole. New body-imaging applications for techniques such as diffusion and spectroscopy are being made possible by faster scan times. Finally, MR-guided intervention is increasing the role of MR imaging further, in tissue diagnosis and the treatment of disease.

References

[1] Martin DR, Friel H, Danrad R, et al. Approach to abdominal imaging at 1.5 Tesla and optimization at 3 Tesla. Magn Reson Imaging Clin N Am 2005;13:241–54.

[2] Merkle EM, Dale BM. Abdominal MRI at 3.0 T: the basics revisited. AJR Am J Roentgenol 2006; 186(6):1524–32.

[3] Morakkabati-Spitz N, Schild HH, Kuhl CK, et al. Female pelvis: MR imaging at 3.0 T with sensitivity encoding and flip-angle sweep technique. Radiology 2006;241(2):538–45.

[4] Bammer R, Schoenberg SO. Current concepts and advances in clinical parallel magnetic resonance imaging. Top Magn Reson Imaging 2004; 15(3):129–58.

[5] Sodickson DK, Manning WJ. Simultaneous acquisition of spatial harmonics: fast imaging with radiofrequency coil arrays. Magn Reson Med 1997;38:591–603.

[6] Griswold MA, Jakob PM, Heidemann RM, et al. Generalized autocalibrating partially parallel acquisitions (GRAPPA). Magn Reson Med 2002; 47:1202–10.

[7] Pruessmann KP, Weiger M, Scheidegger MB, et al. SENSE: sensitivity encoding for fast MRI. Magn Reson Med 1999;42:952–62.

[8] Glockner JF, Hu HH, Stanley DW, et al. Parallel MR imaging: a user's guide. Radiographics 2005; 25(5):1279–97.

[9] Pruessmann KP. Parallel imaging at high field strength: synergies and joint potential. Top Magn Reson Imaging 2004;15(4):237–44.

[10] Caravan P, Lauffer RB, et al. Contrast agents: basic principles. In: Edelman RR, Hesselink JR, Zlatkin MB, editors. Clinical magnetic resonance imaging. 3rd edition. Philadelphia: Saunders Elsevier; 2006. p. 358–76.

[11] Harisinghani MG, Saini S, Weissleder R, et al. MR lymphangiography using ultrasmall superparamagnetic iron oxide in patients with primary abdominal and pelvic malignancies: radiographic-pathologic correlation. AJR Am J Roentgenol 1999;172:1347–51.

[12] Rockall AG, Sohaib SA, Harisinghani MG, et al. Diagnostic performance of nanoparticle-enhanced magnetic resonance imaging in the diagnosis of lymph node metastases in patients with endometrial and cervical cancer. J Clin Oncol 2005;23(12):2813–21.

[13] Choi SH, Moon WK, Hong JH, et al. Lymph node metastasis: ultrasmall superparamagnetic iron oxide-enhanced MR imaging versus PET/CT in a rabbit model. Radiology 2007;242(1): 137–43.

[14] Weissleder R. Scaling down imaging: molecular mapping of cancer in mice. Nat Rev Cancer 2002;2(1):11–8.

[15] Danthi SN, Pandit SD, Li KCP. A primer on molecular biology for imagers: VII. Molecular imaging probes. Acad Radiol 2004;11:1047–54.

[16] Colagrande S, Carbone SF, Carusi LM, et al. Magnetic resonance diffusion-weighted imaging: extraneurological applications. Radiol Med (Torino) 2006;111(3):392–419.

[17] Naganawa S, Sato C, Kumada H, et al. Apparent diffusion coefficient in cervical cancer of the uterus: comparison with the normal uterine cervix. Eur Radiol 2005;15(1):71–8.

[18] Righini A, Bianchini E, Parazzini C, et al. Apparent diffusion coefficient determination in normal fetal brain: a prenatal MR imaging study. AJNR Am J Neuroradiol 2003;24:799–804.

[19] Prayer D, Kasprian G, Krampl E, et al. MRI of normal fetal brain development. Eur J Radiol 2006;57(2):199–216.

[20] Coakley FV, Qayyum A, Kurhanewicz J. Magnetic resonance imaging and spectroscopic imaging of prostate cancer. J Urol 2003;170(6 Pt 2):S69–75.

[21] Tse GM, Cheung HS, Pang LM, et al. Characterization of lesions of the breast with proton MR spectroscopy: comparison of carcinomas, benign lesions, and phyllodes tumors. AJR Am J Roentgenol 2003;181:1267–72.

[22] Buchtal SD, den Hollander JA, Merz NB, et al. Abnormal myocardial phosphorus-31 nuclear magnetic resonance spectroscopy in women with chest pain but normal coronary angiograms. N Engl J Med 2000;342:829–35.

[23] Khan SA, Cox IJ, Hamilton G, et al. *In vivo* and *in vitro* nuclear magnetic resonance spectroscopy as a tool for investigating hepatobiliary disease: a review of 1H and 31P MRS applications. Liver Int 2005;25:273–81.

[24] Cho SG, Lee DH, Lee KY, et al. Differentiation of chronic focal pancreatitis from pancreatic carcinoma by in vivo proton magnetic resonance spectroscopy. J Comput Assist Tomogr 2005; 29(2):163–9.

[25] Katz-Brull R, Rofsky NM, Morrin MM, et al. Decreases in free cholesterol and fatty acid unsaturation in renal cell carcinoma demonstrated by breath-hold magnetic resonance spectroscopy. Am J Physiol Renal Physiol 2005;288:F637–41.

[26] Mahon MM, Williams AD, Soutter WP, et al. 1H magnetic resonance spectroscopy of invasive cervical cancer: an in vivo study with ex vivo corroboration. NMR Biomed 2004;17(1):1–9.

[27] Kok RD, van den Bergh AJ, Heerschap A, et al. Metabolic information from the human fetal brain obtained with proton magnetic resonance spectroscopy. Am J Obstet Gynecol 2001;185(5): 1011–5.

[28] Carrino JA, Jolesz FA, et al. Interventional and intraoperative magnetic resonance imaging. In: Edelman RR, Hesselink JR, Zlatkin MB, editors. Clinical magnetic resonance imaging. 3rd edition. Philadelphia: Saunders Elsevier; 2006. p. 512–40.

[29] Tempany CM, Stewart EA, McDannold N, et al. MR imaging-guided focused ultrasound surgery of uterine leiomyomas: a feasibility study. Radiology 2003;226(3):897–905.

[30] Jacobs MA, Herskovits EH, Kim HS. Uterine fibroids: diffusion-weighted MR imaging for monitoring therapy with focused ultrasound surgery—preliminary study. Radiology 2005; 236(1):196–203.

[31] Stewart EA, Rabinovici J, Tempany CM, et al. Clinical outcomes of focused ultrasound surgery for the treatment of uterine fibroids. Fertil Steril 2006;85(1):22–9.

MAGNETIC
RESONANCE
IMAGING CLINICS

Magn Reson Imaging Clin N Am 14 (2007) 439–453

MR Imaging of Benign Uterine Disease

Michèle A. Brown, MD

MR has become the imaging modality of choice for various benign and malignant gynecologic diseases. For patients who have benign disease, accurate diagnosis can be achieved with fast MR imaging protocols that conserve valuable scanner time. This article describes MR protocols and the typical findings of various benign conditions of the uterine corpus and cervix, including congenital anomalies, leiomyomas, adenomyosis, and complications related to pregnancy.

MR imaging technique

Patients should fast for at least 4 hours before MR imaging of the pelvis and should be asked to void immediately before being positioned on the scan table. An empty bladder helps to reduce breathing-related phase artifact, decrease superior displacement of the uterine fundus where it is often obscured by bowel peristalsis, and increase patient comfort. Optional patient preparation includes antispasmodics such as glucagon (1 mg, intravenously or intramuscularly), to decrease motion artifact related to bowel peristalsis. For cases of suspected cervical or vaginal pathology, intravaginal gel may be used to distend the vaginal fornices and optimize visualization [1]. The patient is placed feet-first on the table in the supine position, and a phased-array torso coil is placed with its superior edge at the level of the iliac crests. For evaluation of the urethra, a smaller phased-array surface coil may be used, centered on the perineum. The use of endoluminal coils is advocated by some investigators for the evaluation of urethral symptoms [2]. The advantages of endoluminal coils include greater spatial resolution, whereas the disadvantages include cost, patient acceptance, and anatomic distortion caused by the presence of the coil. With the increasing availability of high field strength units, another choice is whether to image at 1.5 T or 3 T. This article addresses imaging at 1.5 T; techniques for image optimization at 3 T are discussed in this issue in a separate article by Hussain and colleagues.

Many MR sequences are available for imaging the female pelvis. The optimal imaging protocol provides adequate diagnostic information in a limited amount of time. For this reason, many centers use

Department of Radiology, University of California, San Diego Medical Center, 200 West Arbor Drive, San Diego, CA 92103, USA
E-mail address: m9brown@ucsd.edu

1064-9689/07/$ – see front matter © 2007 Elsevier Inc. All rights reserved.
mri.theclinics.com

doi:10.1016/j.mric.2007.01.006

different approaches for patients who have presumed benign disease and those with malignant disease. For benign disease, fast breath-hold sequences often are adequate despite slightly decreased resolution [3]. Accurate diagnosis can be achieved in minimal scan time using a limited number of breath-hold sequences and no contrast media. One such protocol, illustrated in Fig. 1, involves five separate sequence acquisitions, as follows

1. Large field of view (FOV) coronal T2-weighted single-shot (SS) echo train spin-echo (ETSE), to include the pelvis and lower portion of the kidneys
2. Large FOV axial T2-weighted single-shot ETSE
3. Small FOV oblique sagittal T2-weighted ETSE
4. Small FOV oblique axial T2-weighted ETSE
5. Small FOV oblique axial dual echo T1-weighted gradient echo.

A small FOV of 20 to 24 cm, depending on the imaging plane and size of the patient, helps improve resolution of the normally small structures of the female pelvis. These sequences are angled to either the uterus or the cervix, depending on the clinical question. It is important to plan the oblique sagittal image of the uterus based in the straight axial, because most women have a uterus angled to the left or right [4]. As summarized in Table 1, each sequence in this brief protocol serves a particular purpose, and the combined information is sufficient for the diagnosis of leiomyomas and adenomyosis. Specific additional sequences can be added for indications such as uterine anomalies (angled coronal T2-weighted ETSE of uterus) or known or suspected coexisting disease such as endometriosis (fat saturated T1-weighted gradient echo), or for preprocedural evaluation for uterine artery embolization (UAE) (gadolinium-enhanced T1-weighted gradient echo). Although the exclusive use of breath-hold sequences is sufficient, and serves to minimize the examination time for benign disease, longer protocols are needed for malignant disease. For the evaluation of cancer, described in the subsequent article, longer duration, high-resolution T2-weighted ETSE and postgadolinium fat-suppressed T1-weighted images are needed.

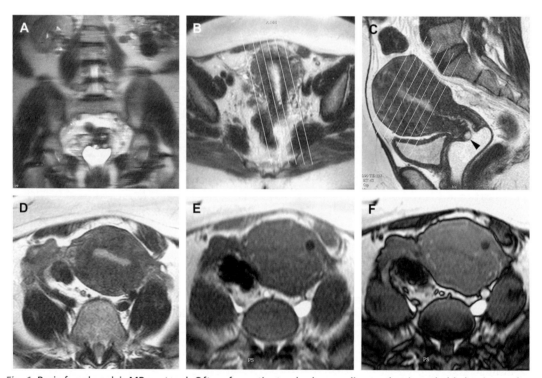

Fig. 1. Basic female pelvis MR protocol. Often, for patients who have a disease that is probably benign, a short examination without contrast is sufficient. Coronal (*A*) and axial (*B*) single-shot echo train spin-echo (SS-ETSE) sequences are performed first using a large FOV of approximately 40 cm. The FOV is reduced for subsequent sequences to 20 to 24 cm, depending on patient size. A sagittal T2-weighted ETSE sequence through the uterus (*C*) is prescribed off the axial SS-ETSE and is used to plan the angled axial T2-weighted ETSE image (*D*) and the gradient echo image obtained as a dual echo to provide in-phase (*E*) and out-of-phase (*F*) T1-weighted images. Note the distension of the vagina with gel, which outlines the cervix and a small nabothian cyst (*arrowhead in C*). Diffuse adenomyosis is present also, with marked thickening of the uterine junctional zone seen best on T2-weighted ETSE images (*C, D*).

Table 1: **Basic MR imaging protocol for benign disease of the uterus and cervix**

Sequence	Purpose
Coronal SS-ETSE	*hydronephrosis, renal anomalies,*
Axial SS-ETSE Oblique sagittal ETSE	*direct oblique sagittal image evaluation of uterus/cervix; direct oblique axial image*
Oblique axial ETSE	*evaluation of uterus/cervix, ovaries*
Oblique axial dual-echo gradient echo	*T1 + chemical shift information*

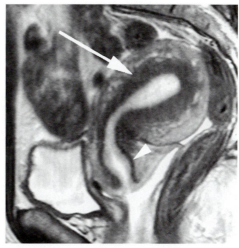

Fig. 2. Zonal anatomy of the uterine corpus and cervix. Sagittal T2-weighted ETSE image of a retroflexed uterus. The central hyperintensity in the uterine corpus represents the endometrium. The band of low signal intensity represents the junctional zone (*arrow*), which appears continuous with the fibrous stroma of the cervix (*arrowhead*). The outer layer of the myometrium is of intermediate signal intensity.

Despite patient fasting, the administration of glucagon, and the use of fast imaging sequences, motion remains a challenge in pelvic imaging, albeit less than for abdominal imaging. Techniques to minimize the effects of patient motion include the placement of a saturation band over the fat in the anterior abdominal wall to minimize artifact on non–fat-suppressed sagittal images and the use of an anteroposterior frequency-encoding direction for axial images.

Normal anatomy

The uterus is divided anatomically into the corpus and the cervix and normally measures 6 to 9 cm long in premenopausal women. The uterine corpus is divided histologically into the outer serosa, the myometrium, and the endometrium. On T1-weighted images, the entire uterus is isointense to muscle, whereas on T2-weighted images, the premenopausal uterus contains three distinct zones: a central high-signal-intensity endometrium and secretions, the middle low-signal-intensity junctional zone, and the outer intermediate-signal-intensity myometrium (**Fig. 2**) [5]. The low-signal-intensity junctional zone represents the innermost layer of the myometrium, which has less water content, more compact smooth muscle, and a greater percentage of nuclear area than the outer myometrium [6]. The normal junctional zone ranges from 2 to 8 mm in thickness [5]. The appearance of the junctional zone may change as a function of sustained myometrial contractions or uterine peristalsis. Sustained contractions are important to recognize and distinguish from leiomyomas or adenomyosis [7].

Transiency over the course of the examination is the most helpful diagnostic feature of a sustained contraction; however, sustained contractions also tend to be more oblong and less well defined than leiomyomata, and exert more mass effect on the endometrium than focal adenomyosis (**Fig. 3**). Uterine peristalsis is a subtler phenomenon that occurs continuously in women of childbearing age. The normal peristaltic wave proceeds cephalad during the proliferative phase and caudal during menstruation. This observation suggests a potential role in disorders of fertility, endometriosis, and dysmenorrhea. Peristalsis has been shown on ultrafast T2-weighted imaging as transient thickening that moves up or down the junctional zone [8,9].

With the extended use of oral contraceptives, the uterus decreases in size, the endometrium becomes thin, the junctional zone becomes less prominent, and the outer myometrium becomes brighter on T2-weighted images [10,11]. After menopause, the uterus decreases in overall size, with the uterine corpus becoming smaller relative to the cervix, and the junctional zone not visualized consistently. In women taking tamoxifen, several endometrial and myometrial changes may be seen, including endometrial proliferation, hyperplasia, polyps, carcinoma, leiomyomas, and adenomyosis [10,12–14].

Uterine enhancement varies with the menstrual cycle. In the early proliferative phase, a thin innermost layer of junctional zone shows the earliest enhancement. During menstruation, the entire junctional zone enhances early [15]. The outer myometrium enhances slightly later, and the endometrium enhances last and most intensely (see Fig. 3) [16].

The cervix also appears uniformly isointense to muscle on T1-weighted images. On T2-weighted sequences, the cervix demonstrates four distinct zones: central hyperintense mucous, high-signal-intensity endocervical mucosa and glands, hypointense fibrous stroma, and outer intermediate-signal-intensity loose stoma. The endocervical canal contains innumerable folds and clefts that inspired the term plicae palmatae because the irregular surface was thought to resemble that of a palm tree. Deep clefts involve layers of fibrous stroma and, occasionally, the appearance may mimic that of a fibrous septum (Fig. 4). After gadolinium administration, the endocervical mucosa enhances rapidly, whereas the stroma shows more gradual enhancement [17,18].

Congenital uterine anomalies

Congenital müllerian duct anomalies exist in approximately 1% of women of reproductive age. The prevalence is far higher among women being evaluated for infertility; reproductive problems occur in 25% of women with uterine anomalies, compared with 10% of all women [19]. These anomalies do not cause primary infertility, but are associated with recurrent miscarriage, premature labor, dystocia, cervical incompetence, and intrauterine growth retardation. Resulting from maldevelopment or nonfusion of the müllerian ducts, müllerian duct anomalies are divided into classes with similar clinical features, prognoses, and treatment. Because treatment options vary considerably, accurate preoperative characterization is critical. MR is currently the imaging modality of choice for the evaluation of these anomalies because it provides accurate evaluation of the external contour and the muscular and fibrous septa with the endometrial canal. Unlike hysterosalpingography, MR imaging can detect rudimentary horns that do not communicate with the main endometrial cavity. When evaluating uterine anomalies, it is necessary to add an additional sequence to the basic protocol described previously, a T2-weighted ETSE oriented coronal to the uterus. In complex cases in which this view is difficult to obtain, a three-dimensional acquisition may be acquired and viewed subsequently in any plane. The large FOV single-shot ETSE is helpful to view the kidneys; because of the proximity of the müllerian and wolffian systems embryologically, uterine anomalies are associated frequently with urinary tract anomalies, particularly renal agenesis or ectopia [20]. According to the modified Buttram and Gibbons classification, uterine anomalies can be divided into seven classes [19,21].

Class I: Segmental agenesis or hypoplasia

These anomalies result from abnormal development of the müllerian ducts and may occur in association with a congenital syndrome or chromosomal defect. MR imaging demonstrates absence of the uterus, cervix, or vagina that often is seen best on sagittal T2-weighted sequences. The most common anomaly of this class is a combined form, as seen in patients who have Mayer-Rokitansky-Küster-Hauser syndrome, which involves vaginal agenesis or hypoplasia, intact ovaries and fallopian tubes, and variable anomalies of the uterus, urinary tract, and skeletal system. Patients typically present with primary amenorrhea [20,22].

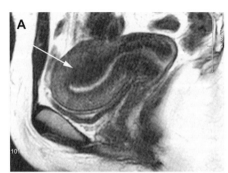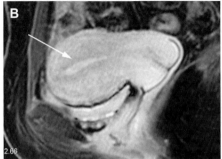

Fig. 3. Uterine contraction. Sagittal T2-weighted ETSE image (*A*) and postgadolinium fat-suppressed T1-weighted gradient echo image (*B*) obtained 35 minutes later. Focal thickening of the junctional zone is seen (*arrow in A*) with mass effect on endometrial canal. After 35 minutes, the contraction is no longer seen. Also note the normal delayed enhancement pattern of the uterus: the endometrium enhances most, followed by the outer myometrium, and the junctional zone is slightly lower signal intensity (*arrow in B*).

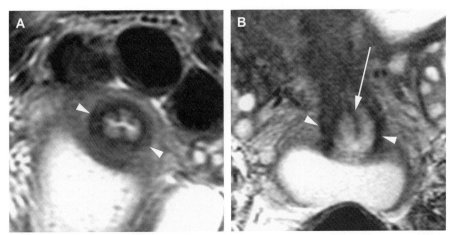

Fig. 4. Normal cervix. T2-weighted ETSE images oriented axial (*A*) and longitudinal (*B*) to the endocervical canal show the cervical zonal anatomy: central hyperintense mucus, high-signal-intensity mucosa and endocervical glands, hypointense fibrous stroma (*arrowheads*), and outer intermediate-signal-intensity loose stroma. Note the irregular inner surface of the fibrous stroma caused by glandular infolding, producing the appearance of septa in some imaging planes (*arrow in B*).

Class II: Unicornuate

Unicornuate uterus results from the maldevelopment of one müllerian duct. On MR images, an elongated uterus is seen with normal zonal anatomy but decreased overall uterine volume. In some cases, incomplete development of the second müllerian duct leads to a rudimentary horn, which may or may not contain endometrium. The identification of this feature is important because endometrium-containing rudimentary horns often are resected surgically to avoid complications. T2-weighted images allow one to detect a hyperintense endometrial stripe within a rudimentary horn and to determine if there is continuity with the main uterine cavity [19,23]. Unicornuate uterus has a particularly high association with renal anomalies, usually renal agenesis.

Class III: Didelphys

Uterus didelphys results from absent fusion of the uterine horns. MR imaging shows two uteri and cervices, often widely divergent (Fig. 5). Vaginal septa may be seen with any uterine anomaly, but is associated most commonly with uterus didelphys. When the septum is oriented transversely, it may obstruct menstrual flow and lead to hematocolpometra. In such cases, MR images show a distended vagina and uterus containing blood products, and a separate normal uterus that is not obstructed [23].

Class IV: Bicornuate

Bicornuate uterus results from incomplete fusion of the uterine horns. On MR imaging, a muscular and fibrous septum separates the uterine horns by more than 4 cm. A fundal indentation more than 1 cm

deep favors bicornuate over septate and is best seen on coronal images of the uterus. The septum of a bicornuate uterus may terminate at the internal os or extend through the cervix, potentially mimicking cervical duplication. Although surgery usually is not necessary, a bicornuate uterus requires a transabdominal approach for repair in symptomatic patients [19,23].

Class V: Septate

Septate uterus occurs because of the failure of resorption of the fibrous septum between the müllerian ducts. Septate uterus is the most common

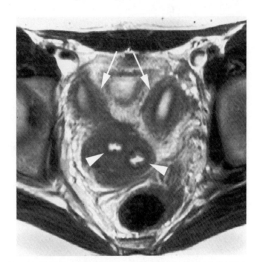

Fig. 5. Uterus didelphys. Axial T2-weighted ETSE image shows complete uterine duplication with two separate, normal-sized corpora (*arrows*); cervices can be seen with two hyperintense endocervical canals (*arrowheads*).

uterine anomaly and has a high association with infertility. A convex, or minimally indented (<1 cm), fundus and a fibrous septum are seen on MR images. Unlike the bicornuate uterus, the uterine horns are separated normally by a distance of 2 to 4 cm [19]. The most important single plane for differentiating a septate from a bicornuate uterus is the coronal image through the uterus (Fig. 6). Accurate distinction is important for management; in symptomatic patients, bicornuate uteri require transabdominal surgical repair, whereas septate uteri can be treated hysteroscopically.

Class VI: Arcuate

Depending on the classification scheme, arcuate uterus is considered a Class VI anomaly or a normal variant. Regardless, this uterine configuration has no definite effect on fertility. On MR images, a short, broad septum is seen that minimally indents the fundal contour of the endometrium.

Class VII: Diethylstilbestrol exposure

Until approximately 30 years ago, diethylstilbestrol was used up to help prevent spontaneous abortion in pregnant women with vaginal bleeding. Uterine anomalies in female children of treated women include hypoplasia, T-shaped uterus, constrictions, and synechiae. In addition, an increased incidence of clear-cell carcinoma of the vagina has been observed. A T-shaped endometrium is seen best on MR images obtained coronal to the endometrium, and constrictions appear as focal thickening of the junctional zone. Hypoplasia of the cervix and uterine cavity may be seen with normal zonal uterine anatomy. Unlike the other classes of uterine

anomalies, diethylstilbestrol-related changes are not associated with urinary tract anomalies [24].

Despite the classification scheme outlined above, these anomalies represent a spectrum of disease, and complex anomalies may show characteristics of multiple classes (Fig. 7) [25]. In fact, because of the difficulty of categorizing complex anomalies, new systems of classification have been proposed [26]. When interpreting MR imaging findings in cases of complex anomalies, it is important to describe the individual components, rather than the class the findings most resemble [19,25,26].

Benign acquired disease of the uterine corpus

Benign disease of the uterine corpus includes endometrial and myometrial processes. Benign endometrial disease includes primary hyperplasia and polyps, whereas benign myometrial disease includes leiomyomas and adenomyosis. The uterine corpus also may be affected by infection, postpartum and postoperative complications, and vascular disease processes such as arteriovenous fistulae.

Endometrial hyperplasia and polyps

Endometrial hyperplasia may occur in postmenopausal women, premenopausal women with polycystic ovary syndrome, or women with estrogen-secreting tumors such as granulosa cell tumors. Endovaginal sonography may reveal endometrial thickening, a nonspecific finding that may be caused by hyperplasia, polyp, carcinoma, or submucosal leiomyoma. Endometrial biopsy is often diagnostic in these cases; however, MR imaging may be helpful if ultrasound is indeterminate and biopsy is limited by difficult anatomy or cervical stenosis. Endometrial polyps also are seen typically in postmenopausal patients, and may be asymptomatic or associated with irregular or persistent bleeding.

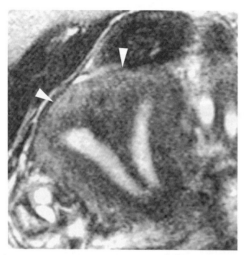

Fig. 6. Septate uterus. T2-weighted ETSE coronal view of the uterus demonstrates a hypointense septum and a convex uterine fundus (*arrowheads*).

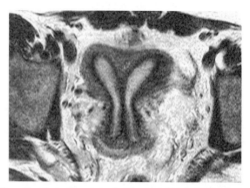

Fig. 7. Complex uterine anomaly. Coronal T2-weighted ETSE image of the uterus shows a slight indentation in the fundus and complete uterine septum, with cervical duplication.

Although malignant transformation into endometrial cancer is seen in less than 1% of cases [27], polyps may coexist with cancer, and biopsy is required to exclude malignancy.

On T2-weighted images, endometrial hyperplasia appears as diffuse thickening of the endometrial stripe, which is isointense or slightly hypointense, compared with normal endometrium. Unfortunately, this appearance is nonspecific and also may be seen with endometrial carcinoma. Endometrial polyps most often appear on T2-weighted images as masses that are isointense, or slightly hypointense, to normal endometrium. MR imaging findings of a fibrovascular stalk or cystic areas favor the diagnosis of polyp over carcinoma or hyperplasia (Fig. 8). Polyps are distinguished readily from submucosal leiomyomas on MR imaging, based on their appearance on T2-weighted images [27]. Polyps typically show pronounced early enhancement that persists on delayed imaging, whereas endometrial carcinoma typically shows only mild enhancement. MR imaging facilitates the differentiation between polyps and endometrial carcinoma; however, biopsy often is still needed because imaging appearances overlap and because carcinomas and polyps may coexist [28].

Leiomyomas

Leiomyomas are common benign tumors that usually are asymptomatic but may lead to various symptoms, the most common of which is abnormal bleeding. Other symptoms are related to mass effect, infertility, second trimester abortions, dystocia, palpable pelvic-abdominal mass, and complication by torsion, infection, acute degeneration, or sarcomatous degeneration [27,29]. Leiomyomas may be classified according to location as submucosal, intramural, subserosal, or cervical. Leiomyomas may be extrauterine also. When symptomatic, leiomyomas may be treated medically, with gonadotropin-releasing hormone analogs; surgically, with hysterectomy or myomectomy; or with minimally invasive techniques such as UAE. More recently, MR-guided focused ultrasound ablation has gained acceptance and shows therapeutic promise [30,31]. The potential advantages of nonsurgical treatment include decreased risk related to surgery and general anesthesia, preservation of fertility, and shorter hospitalization [29,32].

Imaging is used for patients who have suspected leiomyomas to detect, characterize, and localize the tumors. Although ultrasound is used often to establish the diagnosis, MR imaging provides a more accurate determination of the location, number, and degree of degeneration, a feature that is important for selecting patients before minimally invasive treatment. Predictably, degenerated leiomyomas tend to respond poorly to UAE. In addition to aiding patient selection, MR is used to monitor the result of embolization by demonstrating changes in tumor size and enhancement [29,33–36]. MR imaging is valuable also for patients whose ultrasound reveals pedunculated leiomyoma versus solid ovarian mass, to distinguish leiomyomas from adenomyosis, or to visualize the endometrium in a patient with limited ultrasound because of body habitus.

On MR imaging, uterine leiomyomas typically are well circumscribed, isointense to muscle on T1-weighted images, and hypointense on T2-weighted images. A thin hyperintense rim of dilated lymphatic clefts, dilated veins, and edema may be seen on T2-weighted images and helps differentiate leiomyomas from focal adenomyosis (Fig. 9). This rim may enhance with gadolinium administration.

As leiomyomas degenerate, various MR appearances result, such as heterogeneous high signal intensity on T2-weighted images, lack of contrast-enhancement, and, in the case of hemorrhagic (red) degeneration, high signal areas on T1-weighted images [29]. Red degeneration is typical of pregnancy; however, UAE also results in hemorrhagic infarction.

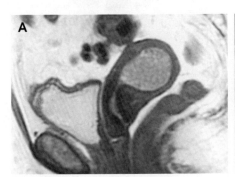
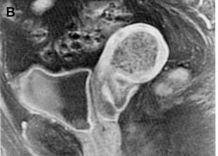

Fig. 8. Endometrial polyp. Sagittal T2-weighted ETSE (*A*) and gadolinium-enhanced fat-suppressed T1-weighted gradient echo (*B*) images show an endometrial mass. On T2-weighted images (*A*), hyperintense cystic spaces are seen within the polyp. On postgadolinium images (*B*), reticular enhancement outlines the cystic foci.

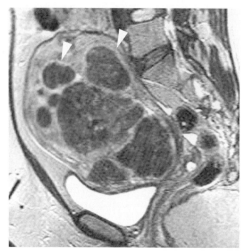

Fig. 9. Multiple uterine leiomyomas. Sagittal T2-weighted ETSE image shows multiple well-defined hypointense masses, some of which have a characteristic thin hyperintense rim (*arrowheads*).

Leiomyomas typically are low in signal intensity on T2-weighted images; however, cellular leiomyomas are a subtype characterized by uniformly high signal intensity, homogeneous enhancement, and good response to embolization. MR imaging not only evaluates tissue enhancement characteristics before embolization but also delineates arterial supply [37,38]. Leiomyomas may parasitize blood supply from other sources, such as ovarian arteries; response to UAE in these cases may be poor (Fig. 10). One of the more common complications of UAE is leiomyoma passage, which often requires no intervention, although hysteroscopic intervention may be indicated if symptoms persist (Fig. 11) [39].

A rare type of leiomyoma is the fat-containing lipoleiomyoma, typically occurring in a subserosal location in perimenopausal women. These benign lesions may present a diagnostic challenge on ultrasound and even on conventional T1- and T2-weighted images. Using dual echo gradient echo sequences or chemically selective fat saturation, the MR diagnosis is straightforward [40].

Among the most useful applications of MR imaging in the female pelvis is in differentiating subserosal leiomyomas from other pelvic masses such as ovarian tumors. A mass that is homogeneously low signal intensity on T2-weighted images is likely to be a leiomyoma, and the main differential of ovarian fibroma is also a benign lesion.

The differentiation of submucosal leiomyomas from endometrial polyps, hyperplasia, or carcinoma usually is possible based on T2-weighted images. An endometrial mass of very low signal intensity on T2-weighted images is likely to be a leiomyoma; however, not all leiomyomas have this characteristic, and overlap may exist between leiomyomas and endometrial polyps or cancer [28].

Malignant degeneration occurs rarely in leiomyomas, and leiomyosarcomas also occur de novo. No MR imaging characteristic has been shown to distinguish benign from malignant uterine smooth muscle tumors consistently. Malignancy should be considered if a leiomyoma enlarges suddenly after menopause or develops indistinct borders; however, the most suggestive finding is evidence of metastatic disease [29].

Adenomyosis

Defined as endometrial stroma and glands within the myometrium, adenomyosis occurs commonly in women of reproductive age and may be microscopic, focal, or diffuse. The condition usually is asymptomatic but may cause pain and abnormal

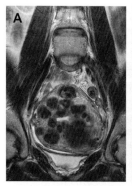
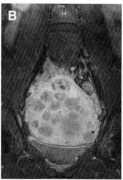
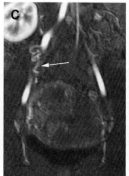
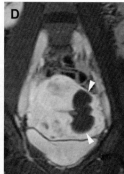

Fig. 10. Unsuccessful UAE caused by recruitment of ovarian artery. Coronal T2-weighted SS-ETSE (*A*) and postgadolinium fat-suppressed T1-weighted gradient echo (*B*) images before embolization, and dynamic gadolinium-enhanced MR angiography (*C*) and delayed postgadolinium fat-suppressed T1-weighted gradient echo (*D*) images after embolization. Multiple enhancing leiomyomas are seen throughout the uterus before the procedure (*A, B*). Postprocedural MR angiogram shows an enlarged right ovary (*arrow in C*). Infarcted leiomyomas are seen on the left (*arrowheads in D*), whereas several right-sided leiomyomas continue to enhance.

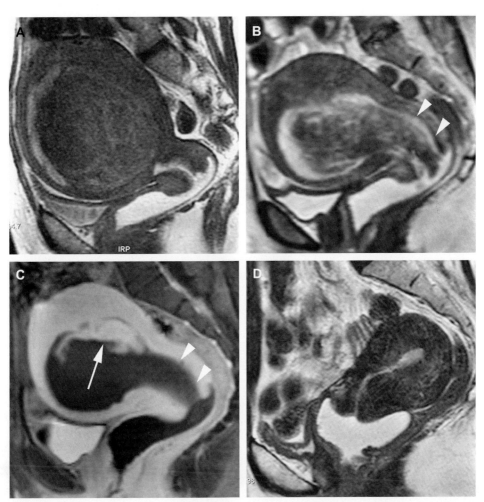

Fig. 11. Passage of a leiomyoma after UAE. Sagittal T2-weighted ETSE image before embolization (*A*), T2-weighted ETSE (*B*) and postgadolinium fat-suppressed T1-weighted gradient echo (*C*) images after embolization, and T2-weighted ESTE image after hysteroscopic resection (*D*). After embolization, spontaneous passage occurred with opening of the cervical os (*arrowheads in B and C*). Residual enhancement is seen (*arrow in C*). After hysteroscopic resection, no fibroid is seen (*D*).

bleeding, usually becoming manifest in perimenopausal women. The term adenomyoma refers specifically to the focal, nodular form of adenomyosis [27,41–44].

Difficult to establish with ultrasound, the diagnosis of adenomyosis versus leiomyomas is important because although leiomyomas can be treated conservatively, hysterectomy currently is considered the definitive treatment for symptomatic adenomyosis [27]. MR imaging is highly accurate; sensitivity and specificity range from 86% to 100% [44]. MR imaging is especially helpful in patients who have coexisting adenomyosis and leiomyomas because ultrasound cannot exclude adenomyosis definitively, and the diagnosis is likely to change treatment considerations.

Adenomyosis is detected on T2-weighted images as thickening of the junctional zone to 12 mm or more, often with punctuate foci of high signal intensity (Fig. 12). Although the junctional zone has been reported to vary from 2 to 8 mm, a lower threshold would have unacceptably large overlap with normal because of sustained myometrial contractions, uterine peristalsis, and diffuse physiologic thickening of the junctional zone during menstruation. Although published data are limited, some investigators have reported normal junctional zone thickness in excess of 12 mm on days 1 and 2 of the menstrual cycle [44]. For this reason, caution should be used when making the diagnosis of adenomyosis based only on junctional zone thickness. Far more reliable is the presence of tiny hyperintense foci on T2-weighted images, a finding considered nearly pathognomonic for adenomyosis. These foci represent small deposits of ectopic endometrium, cystically dilated endometrial glands, or

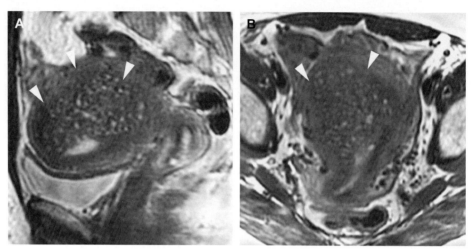

Fig. 12. Focal adenomyosis. Sagittal (*A*) and axial (*B*) T2-weighted ETSE images show a markedly thickened junctional zone in the posterior uterus (*arrowheads*), with sparing of the anterior uterus, where the junctional zone is normal.

hemorrhagic fluid [44]. Tiny, hyperintense foci on T1-weighted images may be seen and may correspond to areas of hemorrhage. If hemorrhage is extensive, cystic adenomyosis can result. MR imaging reveals larger, well-circumscribed, myometrial cysts containing blood products of different ages [43].

Diffuse adenomyosis affecting the entire uterus usually results in uterine enlargement and is more often irregular than smooth in its distribution. Focal adenomyomas are characterized by mass-like thickening of a portion of the junctional zone. Contrast-enhanced sequences may show uniform enhancement [27] or a speckled appearance, with numerous nonenhancing foci corresponding to the punctuate hyperintensities on T2-weighted images.

Focal adenomyosis may mimic leiomyoma, imaging features may overlap, and the two entities often coexist (Fig. 13). Unlike leiomyomas, adenomyomas tend to have poorly defined borders, an elliptic rather than a round shape, and, occasionally, linear striations radiating out from the endometrium [11]. In addition, adenomyomas cause less distortion of the endometrium than leiomyomas of the same size. Myometrial contractions may also have an appearance similar to adenomyosis.

Hysterectomy is the only well-established, definitive treatment for adenomyosis. Success with endometrial ablation, medical therapy with GnRH analogs, and UAE has been observed, but reports of long-term outcome are variable. Patients who have adenomyosis may experience improvement in symptoms after UAE; however, symptoms recur in many patients [36,41,45].

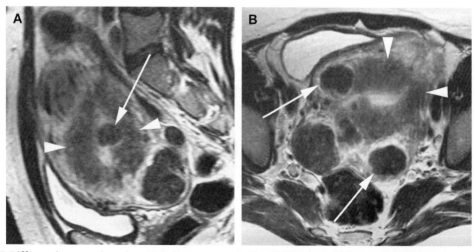

Fig. 13. Diffuse adenomyosis and multiple leiomyomas. Sagittal (*A*) and axial (*B*) T2-weighted ETSE images show a markedly thickened junctional zone (*arrowheads*) with multiple leiomyomas (*arrows*).

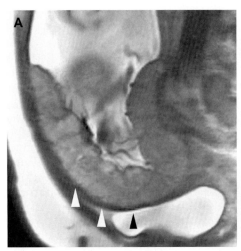
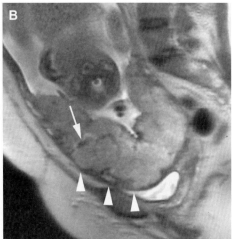

Fig. 14. Noninvasive placenta previa and placenta percreta. Sagittal T2-weighted SS-ETSE images in two different patients who have placenta previa show a normal placenta (*A*) and an invasive placenta (*B*). The normal placenta (*A*) is of moderately high signal intensity, and the inner contour of the third trimester placenta is lobulated in a regular and organized fashion, reflecting cotyledons, whereas the outer contour remains smooth (*arrowheads in A*). In contrast, the invasive placenta (*B*) is more heterogeneous, with distorted internal architecture, dark nonvascular bands (*arrow in B*) and lobulated outer contour (*arrowheads in B*).

Pregnancy-related conditions

Pregnancy predisposes patients to unique pelvic conditions, including invasive placenta, gestational trophoblastic disease, and postpartum complications. MR imaging is well suited to the evaluation of pregnancy-related uterine conditions that may not be as well depicted by ultrasound. Although safety is the most important advantage of MR over CT during pregnancy, superb tissue contrast and anatomic detail also make MR imaging a helpful diagnostic tool for postpartum complications.

Invasive placenta

MR imaging has been used as an adjunct to ultrasound for the evaluation of placenta accreta, which is a leading cause of emergent peripartum hysterectomy. The incidence of invasive placenta is rising, primarily because of an increase in cesarean deliveries. Because of the high maternal morbidity and mortality associated with emergency hysterectomy, it is critical to optimize antenatal diagnosis. Once the diagnosis is made, cesarean section is planned before term, and most women require hysterectomy [46]. Prophylactic internal iliac artery balloons may be placed in attempt to reduce blood loss.

Placenta accreta occurs because of a defect in the decidua basalis that normally prevents villous invasion of the myometrium, and a history of cesarean section is the most common risk factor. Three types are described: placenta accreta vera refers to placental adherence to the myometrium; placenta increta refers to invasion into the myometrium; and placenta percreta refers to invasion through the myometrium to the uterine serosa. Ultrasound identifies placenta previa and often placenta

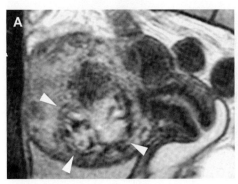
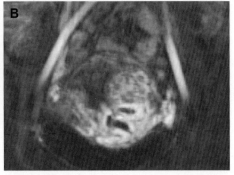

Fig. 15. Gestational trophoblastic disease. Sagittal T2-weighted ETSE image (*A*) and coronal MR angiogram (*B*) show an irregular uterine mass (*arrowheads in A*) indicating myometrial invasion, with marked enhancement in the arterial phase (*B*).

accreta; however, false-positive and false-negative results occur because of maternal vessels or placental position [47,48]. MR imaging is particularly helpful in determining the extent of placental invasion in cases of complex percreta, and has been found to increase diagnostic confidence when ultrasound is suspicious but indeterminate [49].

MR imaging diagnosis depends largely on T2-weighted images obtained as single-shot ETSE, whereas some have found T1- and T2-weighted steady-state gradient echo or dynamic gadolinium-enhanced imaging helpful. On T2-weighted images, the normal placenta is of moderately high signal intensity with regular internal architecture. MR findings suggestive of placental invasion include myometrial thinning, irregularity or focal disruption, dark placental bands on T2-weighted images, disorganized architecture of the placenta, and focal exophytic mass (Fig. 14).

Gestational trophoblastic disease

Gestational trophoblastic disease is a spectrum of conditions including complete or partial hydatidiform mole, invasive mole, and choriocarcinoma. Diagnosis and follow-up of patients who have gestational trophoblastic disease is primarily clinical [50]; however, imaging may be helpful to select patients for adjuvant chemotherapy based on extrauterine invasion, and to evaluate for metastatic disease [51]. On MR imaging, complete moles have been reported to appear as a heterogeneous endometrial mass with cystic spaces, whereas invasive moles and choriocarcinoma involve the myometrium (Fig. 15). Because the trophoblastic

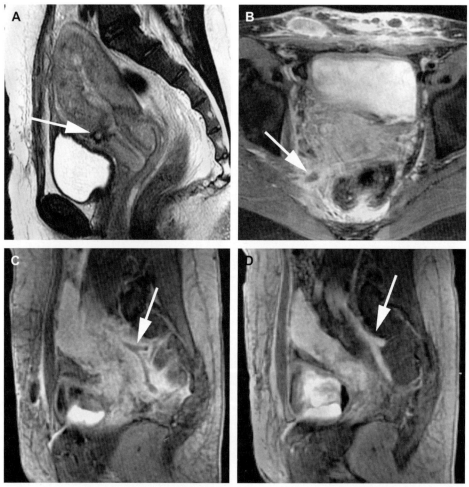

Fig. 16. Postpartum thrombophlebitis. Sagittal T2-weighted ETSE (*A*) and axial (*B*) and sagittal (*C, D*) postgadolinium fat-suppressed T1-weighted gradient echo images in a patient presenting with pulmonary embolism 3 weeks after delivery. The postpartum uterus is enlarged, with indistinct zonal anatomy and evidence of cesarean section (*arrow in A*). Thrombus is seen in the right internal iliac vein (*arrow in B and C*) with surrounding inflammation, whereas the left side is patent (*arrow in D*).

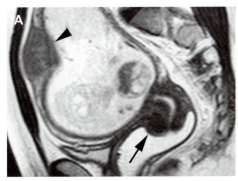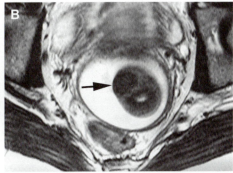

Fig. 17. Cervical leiomyoma. Sagittal (*A*) and transverse (*B*) T2-weighted ETSE images with vaginal gel in a pregnant patient with a suspicious cervical mass on ultrasound. The hypointense round mass in the cervix is consistent with leiomyoma (*arrow in A and B*). A uterine contraction is also seen (*arrowhead in A*).

tissue is highly vascular, early and intense nhancement is seen with gadolinium administration.

Postpartum complications

Postpartum conditions such as infection, venous thromboses, retained products of conception, and hemorrhage are seen well by MR imaging. The normal postpartum uterus is enlarged and lacks distinct zonal anatomy. The junctional zone may not be seen for weeks to months after delivery, and a small amount of free pelvic fluid is considered a normal finding [52]. In cases of postpartum venous thromboses, the diagnosis can be made on MR using flow-sensitive noncontrast sequences or gadolinium enhancement (Fig. 16). In cases of retained products of conception, MR findings reflect the extreme hypervascularity of the residual tissue, which enhances early and avidly with gadolinium, similar to gestational trophoblastic disease. Typically, an overlap in imaging appearance does not cause confusion if the clinical history and beta-human chorionic gonadotropin hormone levels are known. Usually limited to the endometrial canal, retained products of conception have also been reported to appear as a hypervascular mass in the myometrium, similar to acquired uterine arteriovenous fistula. The latter typically results from iatrogenic or pregnancy-related trauma. Arteriovenous fistula is an important diagnosis to consider in a patient who has vaginal bleeding because an attempt to treat with dilatation and curettage could lead to increased bleeding [53].

Benign disease of the cervix

The most common masses encountered in the cervix are nabothian cysts, which are caused by distention of endocervical glands or clefts with mucus. Nabothian cysts rarely are symptomatic, despite growing as large as 4 cm. Variable in signal intensity on T1-weighted images, nabothian cysts typically

are differentiated easily from cervical carcinoma by their well-defined margins and very high signal intensity on T2-weighted images. However, deep nabothian cysts and other benign cervical glandular conditions may have imaging and histologic findings that mimic malignancy [54]. A solid component within or around multiple cysts should raise suspicion for malignancy. Endocervical polyps are also benign cervical masses, and are a common cause of abnormal bleeding. MR may show a cystic or solid polypoid mass in the endocervical canal or vagina [55]. Leiomyomas may also occur in the cervix, and typically are distinguished easily from other cervical masses based on their well-defined margins and low signal intensity on T2-weighted images (Fig. 17).

Summary

MR imaging provides an excellent depiction of various benign conditions of the uterus and cervix. Detection and characterization of leiomyomata and adenomyosis is performed routinely at many centers, and MR plays an important role in stratifying patients into appropriate treatment options. MR imaging is also uniquely well suited to the evaluation of gynecologic conditions that occur during pregnancy and in the postpartum period.

References

[1] Brown MA, Mattrey RF, Stamato S, et al. MRI of the female pelvic using vaginal gel. AJR Am J Roentgenol 2005;185(5):1221–7.

[2] Prasad SR, Menias CO, Narra VR, et al. Cross-sectional imaging of the female urethra: technique and results. Radiographics 2005;25(3):749–61.

[3] Ascher SM, O'Malley J, Semelka RC, et al. T2-weighted MRI of the uterus: fast spin echo vs. breath-hold fast spin echo. J Magn Reson Imaging 1999;9(3):384–90.

[4] Hauth EA, Jaeger HJ, Libera H, et al. MR imaging of the uterus and cervix in healthy women: determination of normal values. Eur Radiol 2007;17(3):734–42.

[5] Lee JK, Gersell DJ, Balfe DM, et al. The uterus: in vitro MR-anatomic correlation of normal and abnormal specimens. Radiology 1985;157:175–89.

[6] Scoutt LM, Flynn SD, Luthringer DJ, et al. Junctional zone of the uterus: correlation of MR imaging and histologic examination of hysterectomy specimens. Radiology 1991;179:403–7.

[7] Togashi K, Kawakami S, Kimura I, et al. Uterine contractions: possible diagnostic pitfall at MR imaging. J Magn Reson Imaging 1993;3: 889–93.

[8] Togashi K, Nakai A, Sugimura K. Anatomy and physiology of the female pelvis: MR imaging revisited. J Magn Reson Imaging 2001;13:842–9.

[9] Kataoka M, Togashi K, Kido A, et al. Dysmenorrhea: evaluation with cine-mode-display MR imaging—initial experience. Radiology 2005; 235(1):124–31.

[10] Fong K, Causer P, Atri M, et al. Transvaginal US and hysterosonography in postmenopausal women with breast cancer receiving tamoxifen: correlation with hysteroscopy and pathologic study. Radiographics 2003;23:137–50.

[11] Ascher SM, Jha RC, Reinhold C. Benign myometrial conditions: leiomyomas and adenomyosis. Top Magn Reson Imaging 2000;14:281–304.

[12] Ascher SM, Johnson JC, Barnes WA, et al. MR imaging appearance of the uterus in postmenopausal women receiving tamoxifen therapy for breast cancer: histopathologic correlation. Radiology 1996;200(1):105–10.

[13] Ascher SM, Imaoka I, Lage JM. Tamoxifen-induced uterine abnormalities: the role of imaging. Radiology 2000;214:29–38.

[14] McCluggage WG, Desai V, Manek S. Tamoxifen-associated postmenopausal adenomyosis exhibits stromal fibrosis, glandular dilatation and epithelial metaplasias. Histopathology 2000;37: 340–6.

[15] Yamashita Y, Harada M, Sawada T, et al. Normal uterus and FIGO stage I endometrial carcinoma: dynamic gadolinium-enhanced MR imaging. Radiology 1993;186:495–501.

[16] Chaudhry S, Reinhold C, Guermazi A, et al. Benign and malignant diseases of the endometrium. Top Magn Reson Imaging 2003;14: 339–57.

[17] DeSouza NM, Hawley IC, Schwieso JE, et al. The uterine cervix on in vitro and in vivo MR images: a study of zonal anatomy and vascularity using an enveloping cervical coil. AJR Am J Roentgenol 1994;163:607–12.

[18] Scoutt LM, McCauley TR, Flynn SD, et al. Zonal anatomy of the cervix: correlation of MR imaging and histologic examination of hysterectomy specimens. Radiology 1993;186:159–62.

[19] Troiano RN, McCarthy SM. Mullerian duct anomalies: imaging and clinical issues. Radiology 2004;233:19–34.

[20] Buttram VC Jr. Mullerian anomalies and their management. Fertil Steril 1943;40:159–63.

[21] The American Fertility Society classifications of adnexal adhesions, distal tubal obstruction, tubal occlusion secondary to tubal ligation, tubal pregnancies, mullerian anomalies and intrauterine adhesions. Fertil Steril 1988;49:944–55.

[22] Reinhold C, Hricak H, Forstner R, et al. Primary amenorrhea: evaluation with MR imaging. Radiology 1997;203:383–90.

[23] Pellerito JS, McCarthy SM, Doyle MB, et al. Diagnosis of uterine anomalies: relative accuracy of MR imaging, endovaginal sonography, and hysterosalpingography. Radiology 1992;183:795–800.

[24] van Gils AP, Tham RT, Falke TH, et al. Abnormalities of the uterus and cervix after diethylstilbestrol exposure: correlation of findings on MR and hysterosalpingography. AJR Am J Roentgenol 1989;153:1235–8.

[25] Pavone ME, King JA, Vlahos N. Septate uterus with cervical duplication and a longitudinal vaginal septum: a mullerian anomaly without a classification. Fertil Steril 2006;85(2):494, e9–10.

[26] Oppelt P, Renner SP, Brucker S, et al. The VCUAM (Vagina Cervix Uterus Adnex-associated Malformation) classification: a new classification for genital malformations. Fertil Steril 2005; 84(5):1493–7.

[27] Hamm B, Kubik Huch RA, Fleige B. MR imaging and CT of the female pelvis: radiologic-pathologic correlation. Eur Radiol 1999;9:3–15.

[28] Grasel RP, Outwater EK, Seigelman ES, et al. Endometrial polyps: MR imaging features and distinction from endometrial carcinoma. Radiology 2000;214:47–52.

[29] Murase E, Siegelman ES, Outwater EK, et al. Uterine leiomyomas: histopathologic features, MR imaging findings, differential diagnosis, and treatment. Radiographics 1999;19:1179–97.

[30] Hindley J, Gedroyc WM, Regan L, et al. MRI guidance of focused ultrasound therapy of uterine fibroids: early results. AJR Am J Roentgenol 2004;183:1713–9.

[31] Stewart EA, Rabinovici J, Tempany CM, et al. Clinical outcomes of focused ultrasound surgery for the treatment of uterine fibroids. Fertil Steril 2006;85(1):22–9.

[32] Siskin GP, Shlansky-Goldberg RD, Goodwin SC, et al. A prospective multicenter comparative study between myomectomy and uterine artery embolization with polyvinyl alcohol microspheres: long-term clinical outcomes in patients with symptomatic uterine fibroids. J Vasc Interv Radiol 2006;17(8):1287–95.

[33] Burn PR, McCall JM, Chinn RJ, et al. Uterine fibroleiomyoma: MR imaging appearances before and after embolization of uterine arteries. Radiology 2000;214:729–34.

[34] Jha RC, Ascher SM, Imaoka I, et al. Symptomatic fibroleiomyomata: MR imaging of the uterus before and after uterine arterial embolization. Radiology 2000;217:228–35.

[35] Pelage JP, Guaou NG, Jha RC, et al. Uterine fibroid tumors: long-term MR imaging outcome after embolization. Radiology 2004;30:803–9.

[36] Jha RC, Takahama J, Imaoka I, et al. Adenomyosis: MRI of the uterus treated with uterine artery embolization. AJR Am J Roentgenol 2003;181:851–6.

[37] Spielmann AL, Keogh C, Forster BB, et al. Comparison of MRI and sonography in the preliminary evaluation for fibroid embolization. AJR Am J Roentgenol 2006;187(6):1499–504.

[38] Kroencke TJ, Scheurig C, Kluner C, et al. Uterine fibroids: contrast-enhanced MR angiography to predict ovarian artery supply—initial experience. Radiology 2006;241(1):181–9.

[39] Spies JB, Spector A, Roth AR, et al. Complications after uterine artery embolization for leiomyomas. Obstet Gynecol 2002;100:873–80.

[40] Ueda H, Togashi K, Konishi I, et al. Unusual appearances of uterine leiomyomas: MR imaging findings and their histopathologic backgrounds. Radiographics 1999;19:131–45.

[41] Pelage JP, Jacob D, Fazel A, et al. Midterm results of uterine artery embolization for symptomatic adenomyosis: initial experience. Radiology 2005;234:948–53.

[42] Byun JY, Kim SE, Choi BG, et al. Diffuse and focal adenomyosis: MR imaging findings. Radiographics 1999;19:161–70.

[43] Reinhold C, Tafazoli F, Mehio A, et al. Uterine adenomyosis: endovaginal US and MR imaging features with histopathologic correlation. Radiographics 1999;19:147–60.

[44] Tamai K, Togashi K, Ito T, et al. MR imaging findings of adenomyosis: correlation with histopathologic features and diagnostic pitfalls. Radiographics 2005;25:21–40.

[45] Kim MD, Kim S, Kim NK, et al. Long-term results of uterine artery embolization for symptomatic adenomyosis. AJR Am J Roentgenol 2007;188(1):176–81.

[46] Oyelese Y, Smulian JC. Placenta previa, placenta accreta, and vasa previa. Obstet Gynecol 2006;107(4):927–41.

[47] Levine D, Hulka CA, Ludmir J, et al. Placenta accreta: evaluation with color Doppler US, power Doppler US, and MR imaging. Radiology 1997;205:773–6.

[48] Maldjian C, Adam R, Pelosi M, et al. MRI appearance of placenta percreta and placenta accreta. Magn Reson Imaging 1999;17:965–71.

[49] Warshak CR, Eskander R, Hull AD, et al. Accuracy of ultrasonography and magnetic resonance imaging in the diagnosis of placenta accreta. Obstet Gynecol. 2006;108(3 Pt 1):573–81.

[50] Wagner BJ, Woodward PJ, Dickey GE. From the archives of the AFIP. Gestational trophoblastic disease: radiologic-pathologic correlation. Radiographics 1996;16:131–48.

[51] Allen SD, Lim AK, Seckl MJ, et al. Radiology of gestational trophoblastic neoplasia. Clin Radiol. 2006;61(4):301–13.

[52] Willms AB, Brown ED, Kettritz UI, et al. Anatomic changes in the pelvis after uncomplicated vaginal delivery: evaluation with serial MR imaging. Radiology 1995;195:91–4.

[53] Kido A, Togashi K, Koyama T, et al. Retained products of conception masquerading as acquired arteriovenous malformation. J Comput Assist Tomogr 2003;27:88–92.

[54] Oguri H, Maeda N, Izumiya C, et al. MRI of endocervical glandular disorders: three cases of a deep nabothian cyst and three cases of a minimal-deviation adenocarcinoma. Magn Reson Imaging 2004;22(9):1333–7.

[55] Okamoto Y, Tanaka YO, Nishida M, et al. MR imaging of the uterine cervix: imaging-pathologic correlation. Radiographics 2003;23:425–45.

MAGNETIC RESONANCE IMAGING CLINICS

Magn Reson Imaging Clin N Am 14 (2007) 455–469

MR Imaging of Malignant Uterine Disease

Michèle A. Brown, MD*, Henrique R. de Abreu, MD

- MR imaging technique
  Endometrial carcinoma
  Uterine sarcoma
  Uterine metastases
  Cervical carcinoma
- Cervical metastases
  Recurrent disease and posttreatment changes
- Summary
- References

MR imaging is used increasingly to image uterine malignancy. It has been shown to be effective for preoperative characterization and staging of endometrial and cervical carcinoma and for the evaluation of posttreatment changes and recurrent disease. This article reviews the MR imaging technique and the imaging characteristics of malignant disease of the uterine corpus and cervix.

MR imaging technique

Benign disease is evaluated adequately with breath-hold sequences only, which minimize examination time; however, the evaluation of cancer necessitates longer duration, high-resolution, T2-weighted and postgadolinium, fat-suppressed, T1-weighted images. Small field-of-view, thin-section images (<5 mm) with high spatial resolution facilitate detection of myometrial and parauterine invasion, and must be oriented to the endometrium or cervical canal. Sequential, postgadolinium, breath-hold, three-dimensional, fast gradient-echo images provide dynamic imaging. Delayed postgadolinium imaging should include high-resolution, non–breath-hold, gradient-echo images, which help detect bladder or rectal wall invasion, delineate fistulas, and differentiate fibrosis from tumor recurrence [1,2].

Motion artifacts from respiration and bowel peristalsis may degrade significantly the critical, long-duration, high-resolution sequences. Although not always necessary for benign disease, certain measures that should be considered in cases of malignancy include the use of anterior saturation bands, the use of glucagon or other antispasmodic agent, and the administration of vaginal gel in cases of suspected cervical disease. Differing techniques of vaginal contrast may be used, but a particularly simple and inexpensive method uses a commercially available surgical lubricant administered by way of a modified suction catheter connected to a 60 mL syringe after the patient is positioned on the scan table [3]. Abdominal wall motion may be decreased by prone positioning. It is particularly important for sequences to be oriented to the uterus or cervix, depending on the structure of interest, to minimize partial volume effects and maximize staging accuracy. High-quality images can be obtained with consistency using a phased-array coil. Endocavitary coils have been found by some to detect parametrial invasion better than a body coil or pelvic phased-array coil [4].

Endometrial carcinoma

The most common gynecologic malignancy, endometrial carcinoma, typically occurs in

Department of Radiology, University of California, San Diego Medical Center, 200 West Arbor Drive, San Diego, CA 92103-8756, USA
* Corresponding author.
E-mail address: m9brown@ucsd.edu (M.A. Brown).

1064-9689/07/$ – see front matter © 2007 Elsevier Inc. All rights reserved.
mri.theclinics.com
doi:10.1016/j.mric.2007.01.007

postmenopausal women, and presents with abnormal bleeding. Most endometrial malignancies are adenocarcinomas, and other types include adenosquamous, clear cell, and papillary serous carcinomas. Adenocarcinomas and adenosquamous carcinomas are graded according to International Federation of Gynecology and Obstetrics (FIGO) definition based on histologic differentiation, whereas clear cell and papillary serous carcinomas, characterized by particularly aggressive behavior, are considered high grade by definition [5]. Prognosis depends on histologic grade (1–3), extension into the cervical stroma, and depth of myometrial invasion, which independently predicts lymph node involvement, recurrence, and 5-year survival.

The presence of deep myometrial invasion correlates well with lymph node invasion [6] and is well-evaluated with MR imaging [7]. The likelihood of myometrial invasion increases with tumor grade, which is used to select patients for lymphadenectomy and specialist referral. The use of MR imaging for preoperative assessment of the myometrium has been shown to improve patient selection for lymphadenectomy for all grades of tumor [8]. For this reason, the routine use of MR imaging is advocated for patients being considered for specialist referral. In addition, MR imaging may be performed in patients who have an established or suspected diagnosis of endometrial cancer in cases of technically limited ultrasound, clinically advanced disease, histologic subtypes that carry poor prognoses, or adenocarcinoma on cervical biopsy that may be either endometrial or cervical in origin. MR imaging also detects cervical stromal involvement, another important prognostic indicator for patients who have endometrial carcinoma.

High-resolution, T2-weighted, and postgadolinium, T1-weighted sequences are critical for the evaluation of endometrial carcinoma. Key imaging planes for the evaluation of myometrial invasion are the short-axis and sagittal views of the uterine corpus. Disruption of the junctional zone indicates invasion. If the junctional zone is not seen distinctly, invasion appears as an irregularity of the endometrial–myometrial interface. The use of dynamic contrast-enhanced sequences improves the assessment of myometrial invasion over T2-weighted images alone [9,10]. The accuracy of MR imaging in differentiating noninvasive from invasive endometrial carcinoma has been reported to range from 69% to 88% [8]. Myometrial invasion has been shown to appear as poorly enhancing regions in the myometrium, continuous with an endometrial mass [11]. Leiomyomas and adenomyosis may also enhance less than normal myometrium, and correlation should be made with T2-weighted images. These benign myometrial

conditions are pitfalls that lead to less accurate staging, whether by MR imaging or pathologic assessment [12]. Over- and understaging may result from these conditions. Stage IA disease may arise in adenomyosis, with or without an associated endometrial tumor. Histologically, endometrial carcinoma involving adenomyosis is not considered invasive if endometrial stoma is seen consistently between the tumor cells and the myometrium [13]. Another pitfall is invasion at the cornua, which is difficult to evaluate because of normal myometrial thinning in this region [12].

FIGO stage 0 (carcinoma in situ) tumors may be undetectable on MR imaging, or appear as endometrial thickening with an intact junctional zone. Poor enhancement of the endometrium may be seen on delayed postgadolinium images.

Stage I tumors are confined to the uterine corpus (Box 1). Noninvasive FIGO stage IA lesions may be undetectable, or appear as endometrial thickening. In some cases, a heterogeneous mass with areas of high and low signal intensity distending the endometrial cavity may be noted, although this finding is nonspecific and also seen with polyps and hyperplasia. An intact junctional zone indicates FIGO stage IA disease that is limited to the endometrium [14]. In patients who have stage IA disease and a poorly delineated junctional zone, the endometrial–myometrial interface appears smooth (Fig. 1). The depth of myometrial invasion is divided into superficial (<50% myometrial thickness, or stage IB), and deep (>50% myometrial thickness, or stage IC). In patients who have myometrial invasion, the junctional zone is interrupted or has an irregular interface with the endometrium (Fig. 2) [11].

Box 1: International Federation of Gynecology and Obstetrics staging of endometrial carcinoma

Stage I: Limited to uterine corpus
IA Endometrium
IB <50% Myometrium
IC >50% Myometrium

Stage II: Extension to cervix
IIA Endocervical glands
IIB Cervical stroma

Stage III: Extension beyond uterus
IIIA Uterine serosa, adnexa, positive peritoneal cytology
IIIB Vagina
IIIC Pelvic or para-aortic lymph nodes

Stage IV: Extension to bladder, rectum, beyond true pelvis
IVA Bladder or rectal mucosa
IVB Distant metastases

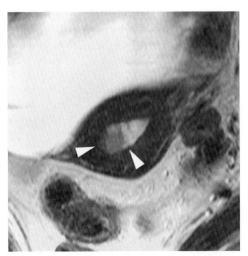

Fig. 1. Endometrial carcinoma without myometrial invasion. T2-weighted echo train spin-echo image axial to the uterus shows a heterogeneous mass widening the endometrial cavity. The endometrial–myometrial interface is smooth and intact (*arrowheads*).

Stage II disease (cervical extension) is characterized by a widening of the internal os on MR images [11]. Superficial extension of endometrial carcinoma to the cervical mucosa (FIGO stage IIA) is seen best on sagittal T2-weighted images by widening of the os with preservation of the cervical fibrous stroma (Fig. 3). However, protrusion into the cervical canal without mucosal invasion may also occur, leading to overstaging by MR imaging [12]. FIGO stage IIB disease is diagnosed when hypointense cervical stroma is disrupted by the relatively hyperintense tumor mass. Dynamic, gadolinium-enhanced, T1-weighted images may show disruption of the normal early mucosal enhancement extending from the endocervical canal outward into the stroma [15]. The accuracy of MR imaging in the diagnosis of cervical invasion has been estimated at 92% [7]. Diagnosis of stromal invasion of the cervix is demonstrated best on oblique axial images angled to the cervix [16]. Because imaging is oriented to the uterine corpus for evaluation of endometrial cancer, the most accurate staging evaluation requires additional sequences if cervical involvement is present. Parametrial invasion, seen as a tumor disrupting the fibrous stroma and extending into surrounding fat, is important to detect because it indicates at least stage IIB disease and has a poor prognosis, requiring more extensive surgery [17,18].

Stage III disease indicates extension outside the uterus and cervix, but limited to the true pelvis. Stage IIIA may appear as full thickness myometrial invasion with uterine contour changes, or a suspicious ovarian mass. The ovaries may be involved either by contiguous spread or metastases, and should be suspected if any indeterminate lesion is noted within the ovary. Invasion of the vagina indicates stage IIIB disease, and enlarged pelvic or para-aortic lymph nodes suggest stage IIIC disease (Fig. 4). Accuracy for detecting malignancy in lymph nodes is poor using CT or MR imaging

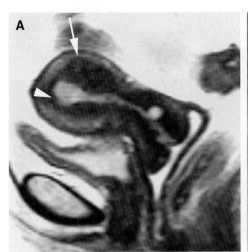
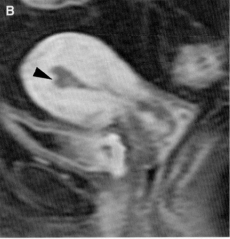

Fig. 2. Endometrial carcinoma stage IB and adenomyosis. Sagittal T2-weighted echo train spin-echo (*A*) and gadolinium-enhanced, fat-suppressed, T1-weighted gradient-echo (*B*) images show endometrial thickening and focal disruption of the inner myometrium anteriorly (*arrowheads*). The junction zone is thickened posteriorly, consistent with adenomyosis (*arrow, A*). Gadolinium-enhanced images are particularly helpful if the junction zone is indistinct, as it may be in postmenopausal women, or abnormal, because of coexisting benign disease such as adenomyosis and leiomyomas.

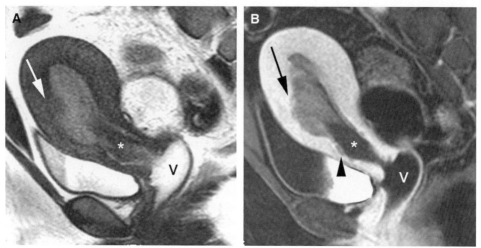

Fig. 3. Endometrial carcinoma stage IIA. Sagittal T2-weighted echo train spin-echo (*A*) and gadolinium-en-hanced, fat-suppressed, T1-weighted, gradient-echo (*B*) images shows endometrial carcinoma asymmetrically widening the endometrial canal. In addition to myometrial invasion (*arrow*), the internal os widens, indicating cervical involvement and stage II disease. In the cervix, the tumor is superficial, with no invasion of cervical stroma (*arrowhead*). Nonenhancing blood products are seen in the cervical canal (*). The vagina (v) is distending with gel in this case to optimize evaluation of cervical and vaginal extension.

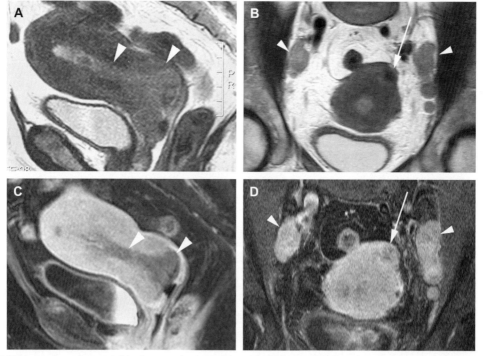

Fig. 4. High-grade endometrioid adenocarcinoma with extension to pelvic lymph nodes. Sagittal (*A*) and trans-verse (*B*) T2-weighted echo train spin-echo and sagittal (*C*) and transverse (*D*) postgadolinium, fat-suppressed, T1-weighted, gradient-echo images. A large mass apparently centered in the cervix widens the endometrial canal and invades the cervical stroma (*arrowheads; A, C*). Surgicopathologic correlation indicated endometrial carcinoma, stage IIIc, with metastatic pelvic lymph nodes (*arrowheads; B, D*). A small leiomyoma is seen in the posterior uterus (*arrow; B, D*).

because size remains the main criterion. Nodes exceeding 1.0 cm short-axis diameter are considered pathologic [19]. Signal intensity characteristics have not been useful in differentiating metastatic from hyperplastic lymphadenopathy in the pelvis. The administration of lymph node–specific contrast agents (ultrasmall superparamagnetic iron oxide) is a promising new approach to improving MR accuracy in lymph node staging [20].

Stage IV disease is present if the tumor spreads to the bladder or rectal mucosa, or if distant metastases involve abdominal or inguinal lymph nodes. Ascites may also be present in advanced disease.

Uterine sarcoma

About 4% of primary uterine cancers are sarcomas. The four subtypes are malignant mixed mullerian tumor, leiomyosarcoma, endometrial stromal sarcoma, and adenosarcoma. The most common is mixed mullerian tumor, also called carcinosarcoma, which has carcinomatous and sarcomatous features and is considered by some to represent a metaplastic carcinoma rather than a sarcoma [21]. Leiomyosarcoma, the second most common subtype, may arise de novo or from malignant degeneration of a benign leiomyoma. Endometrial stromal sarcoma is the third most common, and is further divided into low-grade and high-grade subtypes that each have a distinct presentation and clinical course.

Uterine sarcomas tend to invade blood vessels, lymphatics, and adjacent pelvic organs. Hematogenous metastasis may occur, most commonly to the lungs. Although reports have described the appearance of sarcomas [21–25], MR imaging findings are not specific. MR features that favor sarcoma over endometrial carcinoma include large size, heterogeneous signal with hemorrhage and necrosis, areas of marked delayed enhancement, and invasive or metastatic disease at the time of diagnosis (Fig. 5) [22]. MR cannot differentiate leiomyosarcomas reliably from benign leiomyomas or those pathologically characterized as smooth muscle tumors of uncertain malignant potential. Features that raise concern are large tumor size in an older patient, rapid growth, and ill-defined margins. Other suspicious MR findings that have been described include high signal on T2-weighted images in more than 50% of the tumor, high signal foci on T1-weighted images, and nonenhanced areas (Fig. 6) [25]. Because overlap exists, benign leiomyomas may exhibit some of these characteristics as well (Fig. 7).

Uterine metastases

Involvement of the uterus by nonuterine primary cancer is uncommon and usually occurs by direct extension. Rarely, malignancies spread to the uterus hematogenously or by lymphatics. Uterine metastasis is suggested by the finding of uterine enlargement in a patient who has known metastatic cancer [26].

Cervical carcinoma

Cervical carcinoma is the third most common gynecologic malignancy and is a leading cause of cancer death in women worldwide. Approximately 80% of new cases occur in developing countries. Since the

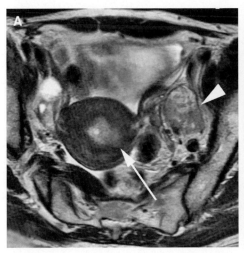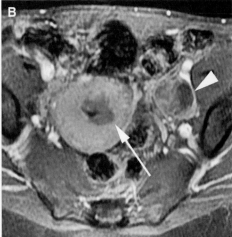

Fig. 5. Uterine carcinosarcoma. Axial T2-weighted echo train spin-echo (*A*) and postgadolinium, fat-suppressed, T1-weighted, gradient-echo (*B*) images show a mildly enhancing endometrial mass with myometrial invasion (*arrow*) and a large metastatic lymph node (*arrowhead*). Lung metastases were also seen at the time of initial presentation.

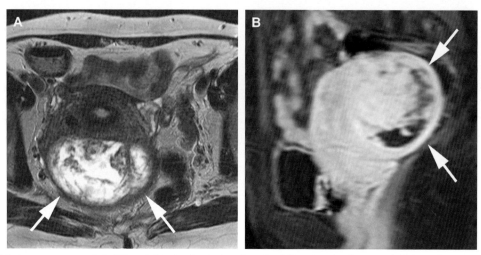

Fig. 6. Leiomyosarcoma. Axial T2-weighted echo train spin-echo (*A*) and sagittal postgadolinium, fat-suppressed, T1-weighted, gradient-echo (*B*) images show a large heterogeneous uterine tumor arising from the posterior myometrium (*arrows*).

routine use of screening with the Papanicoulaou smear, the frequency of, and mortality from, this disease have declined significantly in developed nations. Vaccines against oncogenic human papillomaviruses may reduce the incidence further and could lead to a significant decrease in cervical cancer deaths throughout the world [27]. The Pap smear is most sensitive for squamous cell carcinomas. In addition to a decrease in the incidence of cervical cancer because of screening programs, there has been a relative increase in adenocarcinomas, which carry an overall poorer prognosis. Currently, approximately 85% percent of cervical carcinomas are squamous cell carcinomas and the remaining 15% are adenocarcinomas, adenosquamous carcinomas, undifferentiated carcinomas, and sarcomas. Other than cell type, unfavorable prognostic indicators include young age or advanced stage at diagnosis, lymphadenopathy, lymphovascular invasion, tumor size more than 4 cm, and stromal invasion greater than 5 mm deep.

Extracervical disease occurs by direct extension and by lymphatics. The most commonly involved lymph nodes are in the external iliac, obturator, common iliac, and internal iliac chains. Para-aortic lymph node involvement is seen with tumor extension to the pelvic sidewall or vagina, and inguinal lymph node involvement is seen with extension to the lower vagina. Hematogenous spread, usually to the liver or lung, is rare, and occurs only in the presence of advanced disease.

Cervical carcinoma is staged clinically according to the FIGO staging system (Box 2) [28]. Preoperative assessment of the tumor stage influences the prognosis and choice of treatment. Surgical options

in patients who have small cervical cancer range from conization for carcinoma in situ (FIGO stage 0) to simple hysterectomy, to radical hysterectomy, and lymphadenectomy. Usually, patients who have FIGO stage IA are treated with simple hysterectomy or fertility-preserving surgery, such as trachelectomy. Patients who have invasive carcinoma (FIGO stage IB) or tumor extending to the upper vagina (FIGO stage IIA) may be treated with radical hysterectomy and pelvic lymph node dissection or radiation therapy [29]. Intracavitary brachytherapy is used as an adjunct to surgery for tumors larger than 2 cm, whereas tumors smaller than 2 cm and confined to the cervix may be treated with trachelectomy and lymphadenectomy, if fertility preservation is desired [30]. MR imaging has been found to be helpful in predicting the feasibility of fertility-preserving surgery [31]. Higher-stage cervical cancer (stage IIB and greater) is treated with chemoradiation, which has been shown to have greater disease-free survival, compared with radiation therapy alone [32].

The FIGO staging system has well-known limitations. Significant clinical staging errors have been reported, and important prognostic factors, such as lymphadenopathy, large tumor volume, and tumor extension to the uterine corpus, are not included. Imaging is used to aid staging of cytologically proven disease, and MR is the imaging modality of choice. Compared to CT, MR imaging provides a more accurate assessment of the depth of stromal and parametrial invasion and tumor size [33,34]. A cost-effectiveness study demonstrated significant cost savings with MR imaging, compared with traditional evaluation [35]. Patients

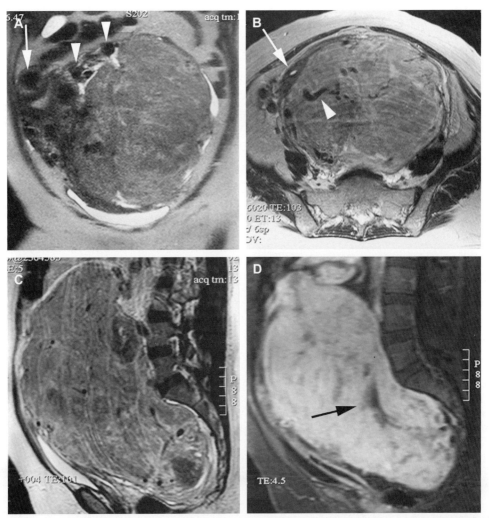

Fig. 7. Benign leiomyoma. Coronal, T2-weighted, single-shot echo train spin-echo (*A*), axial (*B*), and sagittal (*C*) T2-weighted ETSE, and sagittal postgadolinium, fat-suppressed, T1-weighted, gradient-echo (*D*) images show a large irregular mass arising from the pelvis deviating the uterus, which contains a small typical-appearing leiomyoma in the fundus (*arrow, A*). Prominent bridging vessels (*arrowheads, A*) suggest uterine origin, and the deviated uterus with normal endometrium is seen (*B, arrow*). The mass is intermediate in signal intensity of T2-weighted images with large internal flow voids (*arrowheads, B*) and enhances fairly homogeneously with a small area of nonenhancement (*arrow, D*).

who have tumors larger than 2 cm in size, or tumors located entirely within the endocervical canal, have been shown to benefit most from MR imaging [35]. MR imaging is particularly useful in patients who have biopsy-proved adenocarcinoma (endometrial versus cervical in origin), coexistent pelvic masses, and pregnancy at the time of diagnosis.

On MR imaging, oblique, T2-weighted images oriented transverse to the cervical canal are critical, and have been shown to improve staging accuracy [36]. In addition to these true axial images of the cervix, a true coronal sequence may be helpful. Cervical carcinoma appears slightly hypointense to

normal endometrium, and hyperintense to myometrium and cervical stroma. On postgadolinium, fat-suppressed, T1-weighted images, cervical carcinoma enhances less than the adjacent cervical stroma on delayed images. Contrast-enhanced images have not been found to improve the evaluation of parametrial invasion significantly [12].

FIGO stage I disease is restricted to the cervix. Stage IA disease may not be visible, whereas stage IB disease is seen as a high signal intensity mass on T2-weighted images surrounded by preserved hypointense cervical stroma (Fig. 8). Even large tumors may be limited to the cervix; a completely

Box 2:   International Federation of Gynecology and Obstetrics staging of cervical carcinoma

Stage 0: Carcinoma in situ

Stage I: Limited to cervix
IA Microinvasion
IB Clinically invasive
　　IB1 < 4 cm
　　IB2 > 4 cm

Stage II: Extension beyond cervix
IIA Upper two thirds of vagina
IIB Parametrium

Stage III: Lower vagina, pelvic sidewall, ureter
IIIA Lower third of vagina
IIIB Pelvic sidewall or ureteral obstruction

Stage IV: Extension to bladder, rectum, beyond true pelvis
IVA Bladder or rectal mucosa
IVB Distant metastases

intact ring of low signal intensity cervical stroma helps exclude parametrial invasion and is best seen on images oriented axial to the cervix (Fig. 9).

A tumor is classified as stage IIA when it invades the upper two thirds of the vagina. Disruption of the low signal intensity vaginal wall, or the presence of a thickened hyperintense vagina, indicate tumor invasion. An important criterion for management is the presence or absence of parametrial invasion, which indicates FIGO stage IIB disease. Parametrial

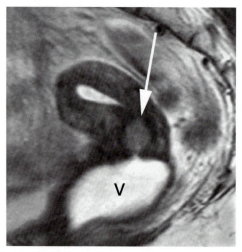

Fig. 8. Cervical carcinoma stage IB1. Sagittal T2-weighted echo train spin-echo image shows a small endocervical mass (*arrow*) surrounded by intact fibrous stroma. The tumor has high signal intensity relative to the cervical stroma and myometrium. Gel was used to distend the vagina (v).

extension is diagnosed by areas of complete disruption of the cervical stroma, often associated with irregularity or stranding within the parametrial fat (Fig. 10).

In FIGO stage IIIA disease, tumor mass extends to the lower third of the vagina, often seen best on sagittal T2-weighted images (Fig. 11). Because of the lymphatic drainage of the distal vagina, enlarged inguinal nodes may be seen with distal vaginal invasion. Infiltration of the pelvic wall, or obstruction of one or both ureters, corresponds to stage IIIB disease. Pelvic sidewall invasion is suggested when the normal low signal intensity of the levator ani, pyriformis, or obturator internus muscle is disrupted on T2-weighted images.

Invasion of the urinary bladder or rectal wall (stage IVA) is suspected when the normally present fat planes between the organs are obliterated. Furthermore, a hyperintense disruption of the otherwise hypointense urinary bladder or rectal wall on T2-weighted images might be seen, and a nodular wall thickening or intraluminal masses may be present [37]. Contrast-enhanced images are also useful in cases of suspected invasion of the bladder or rectum, or if the tumor volume is large and necrotic areas or fistulas are suspected, particularly in the postradiation setting [37–39]. For bladder invasion, the interruption of the hypointense wall on MR imaging is more accurate than on CT, but the modalities have been found to be similar for rectal invasion [34]. Using MR imaging, contrast-enhanced images appear to be superior to T2-weighted images for bladder or rectal wall invasion [38].

Lymph node metastases are not part of FIGO staging but do affect prognosis and treatment decisions. The accuracy of detecting lymph node metastases based on size is poor. Although not always present, central necrosis of a lymph node has been shown to be more accurate than size in predicting malignancy [40]. Others have reported that spiculated or lobulated shape is predictive of metastasis [41]. Developments such as lymph node–specific contrast agents and sentinel node mapping may improve lymph node management in gynecologic tumors [20,42].

Adenocarcinoma, undifferentiated carcinoma, and sarcoma

The relative incidence of adenocarcinoma and its variations has increased over the past several decades, and it is associated with a worse prognosis than squamous cell carcinoma. Because up to 30% of cervical adenocarcinomas have endometrioid elements, pathologic differentiation from endometrial carcinoma may be difficult [43]. In patients who have adenocarcinoma diagnosed by

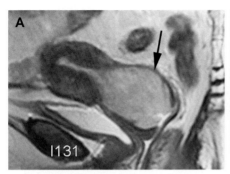
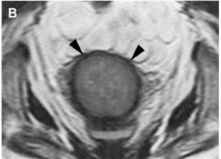

Fig. 9. Cervical adenocarcinoma stage IB2. Sagittal (*A*) and oblique axial (*B*) T2-weighted echo train spin-echo images. A tumor (*arrow, A*) of intermediate signal is seen within the cervix. The tumor is surrounded entirely by normal hypointense cervical stroma (*arrowheads, B*), excluding parametrial invasion.

cervical biopsy, MR imaging may reveal the origin and guide proper management. MR features that favor endometrial origin include endometrial thickening or distension by a mass, invasion of the myometrium directly from the endometrium, and the presence of a complex ovarian mass. If myometrial invasion is seen from the region of the cervix only, the origin is likely cervical (see Fig. 9). However, some tumors have an intermediate appearance, and it is not possible to determine tumor origin based on MR imaging appearance (see Fig. 4). Adenosquamous carcinoma has a worse prognosis than either squamous cell carcinoma or adenocarcinoma (Fig. 12) [44].

Adenoma malignum (also called minimal deviation adenocarcinoma) is a rare subtype of mucinous adenocarcinoma, composing about 3% of cervical adenocarcinomas, and is associated with Peutz-Jeghers syndrome [45]. It carries a poor prognosis and classically presents with the nonspecific symptom of watery discharge. The MR imaging appearance of adenoma malignum has been described as a multicystic mass that extends from the endocervix into the cervical stroma. The mass typically has solid enhancing components that help differentiate it from benign nabothian cysts, but in some cases it is not possible to distinguish malignancy from cervical hyperplasia, polyps, or other benign cystic lesions [43,45,46]. An unusual cervical neoplasm is adenosarcoma, a variant of mixed mesodermal tumor that usually occurs in the endometrium. Cervical adenosarcomas may present with vaginal bleeding and have the gross appearance of a benign polyp (Fig. 13) [47].

Cervical cancer diagnosed during pregnancy

Cervical cancer occurs once in every 1200 to 10,000 pregnancies [48]. Although uncommon, the diagnosis of cervical carcinoma during pregnancy raises difficult management issues. Because clear-cut treatment guidelines do not exist, management is individualized, based on stage of disease, gestational age, and desire for the pregnancy. With close surveillance, deliberate delay of therapy to achieve fetal lung maturity is an option for early-stage cancer (stage IA1, stromal invasion <3 mm deep and

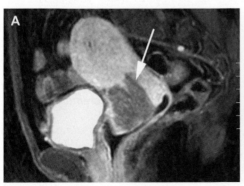
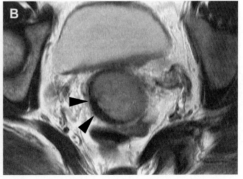

Fig. 10. Cervical carcinoma stage IIB. Sagittal postgadolinium, fat-suppressed, T1-weighted, gradient-echo (*A*) and oblique axial, T2-weighted echo train spin-echo (*B*) images show a large cervical tumor that enhances less than cervical stroma on delayed images (*arrow, A*). Normal hypointense cervical stroma is seen on the right posteriorly (*arrowheads, B*) but is disrupted on the left where the tumor extends to the parametrium.

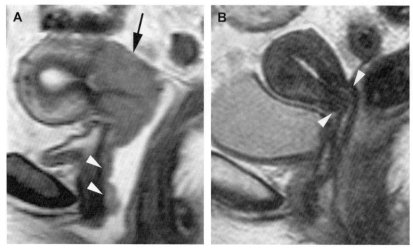

Fig. 11. Cervical carcinoma with vaginal extension, before and after pelvic irradiation. Sagittal T2-weighted echo train spin-echo before treatment (*A*) and after treatment (*B*) show hyperintense cervical carcinoma (*arrow, A*) with extension to the vagina (*arrowheads, A*), which is distended partially with vaginal gel. After radiation therapy, the mass is not seen and the size of the cervix (*arrowheads, B*) and the uterine corpus are decreased markedly.

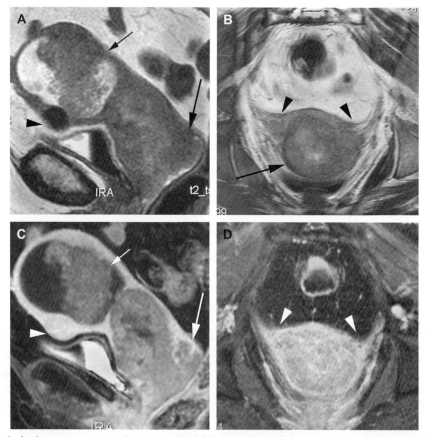

Fig. 12. Cervical adenosquamous carcinoma. Sagittal (*A*) and oblique (*B*) T2-weighted echo train spin-echo and sagittal (*C*) and oblique (*D*) postgadolinium, fat-suppressed, T1-weighted, gradient-echo images show a large mass in the cervix extending from the inferior cervix (*large arrow; A, C*) to the endometrium (*small arrow; A, C*). A small leiomyoma is seen in the anterior uterus (*arrowhead; A, C*). Oblique images oriented axial to the cervix show a small region of intact fibrous stroma (*arrow, B*) and extensive parametrial invasion, with involvement of the uterosacral ligaments (*arrowheads; B, D*).

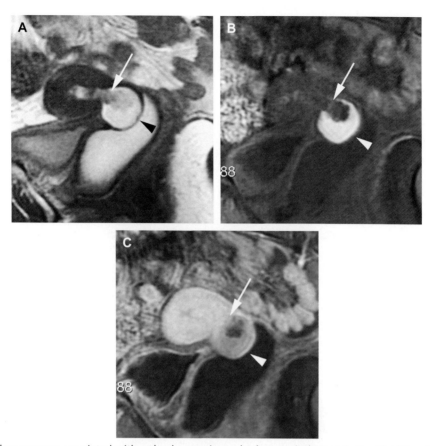

Fig. 13. Adenosarcoma associated with polyp in a patient who has cervical stenosis. Sagittal T2-weighted echo train spin-echo (*A*) and fat-suppressed, T1-weighted, gradient-echo images before (*B*) and after (*C*) gadolinium show a polypoid mass (*arrow*) in the cervix, which is distended by blood caused by stenosis at the external os (*arrowhead*), which, in this case, is seen outlined by vaginal gel. Portions of the lesion enhance with contrast (*arrow, C*). Resection of the polyp revealed low-grade adenosarcoma; a subsequent hysterectomy revealed no additional disease.

<7 mm wide) without histologic evidence of lymphovascular space invasion [48,49]. MR is well-suited to evaluating pregnant patients who have cervical carcinoma because it allows estimation of tumor volume, and depicts extrauterine spread and metastatic disease without ionizing radiation (Fig. 14).

Cervical metastases

The cervix is an uncommon site for metastatic disease, but it may be involved occasionally by direct extension from bladder or colorectal cancer. Hematogenous or lymphatic metastases rarely reach the cervix.

Recurrent disease and posttreatment changes

After completion of treatment of endometrial or cervical cancer, patients undergo clinical and imaging surveillance for recurrence. Early detection is important because prompt additional treatment by chemotherapy or radiation therapy may improve prognosis. Most recurrence occurs within 2 years of treatment, and common sites include the vaginal cuff, the perirectal fascia, the pelvic and retroperitoneal lymph nodes, and the pelvic sidewall. Less commonly, liver, bone, or peritoneal recurrence is seen [50]. On T2-weighted images, local recurrence is more often hyperintense, whereas fibrosis is more often hypointense, although soon after radiotherapy, parametrial invasion may be overestimated because of similar signal intensities of tumor and surrounding edema [51]. Delayed enhancement of the cervix after gadolinium is nonspecific and can be observed in recurrent tumor and postradiation fibrosis, inflammation, and radiation necrosis [52]. On dynamic contrast-enhanced images, recurrence enhances earlier than fibrosis [53]. Gadolinium-enhanced imaging is helpful in demonstrating parametrial and pelvic sidewall recurrence.

Irradiation of the uterus in premenopausal patients results in a decrease in the size of the uterine

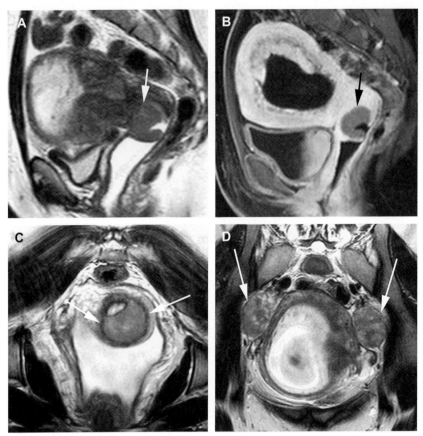

Fig. 14. Cervical cancer diagnosed during pregnancy, stage IB. Sagittal T2-weighted echo train spin-echo (*A*) and gadolinium-enhanced, fat-suppressed, T1-weighted, gradient-echo (*B*), and oblique axial T2-weighted echo train spin-echo (*C, D*) images show a mass confined to the cervix (*arrow; A, B*) surrounded by an intact ring of fibrous stroma (*arrows, C*). Large metastatic pelvic lymph nodes (*arrows, D*) do not affect staging but do affect prognosis and management.

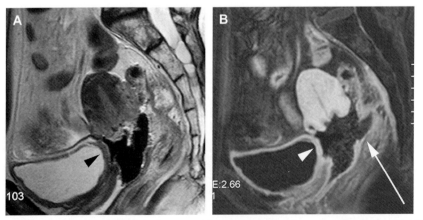

Fig. 15. Large cervical cancer after radiation therapy with necrosis and rectovaginal fistula. Sagittal T2-weighted echo train spin-echo (*A*) and postgadolinium, fat-suppressed, T1-weighted, gradient-echo (*B*) images show necrosis of the cervix. The bladder wall is thickened (*arrowhead*) and, posterior to the bladder, the vaginal wall and anterior rectal wall are disrupted completely. A large communication is seen between the rectum and vagina (*arrow, B*) with stool in the vaginal vault.

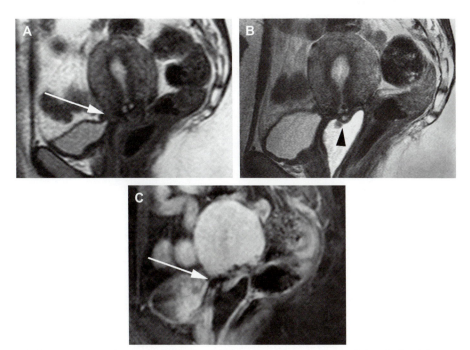

Fig. 16. Trachelectomy. Sagittal T2-weighted echo train spin-echo images before (*A*) and after (*B*) administration of vaginal gel, and sagittal postgadolinium, fat-suppressed, T1-weighted, gradient-echo (*C*) images show absence of the cervix (*arrow*, *A*). After distension of the vagina, irregularity at the surgical margin is apparent (*arrowhead*, *B*). Suture artifact is well seen on gradient-echo images (*arrow*, *C*).

corpus and cervix, thinning of the endometrium, a decreased signal intensity of the myometrium, and loss of uterine zonal anatomy on T2-weighted sequences (see Fig. 11). These changes likely reflect a combination of the direct radiation effects on the uterus and the loss of hormonal stimulation from ovarian function suppression. Late changes include fibrosis, tissue necrosis, and, in some cases, fistula formation (Fig. 15). Postgadolinium, fat-suppressed, T1-weighted images are most helpful to delineate small fistulae.

Radical trachelectomy is a fertility-preserving treatment for early-stage cervical cancer. Usually performed transvaginally in association with laparoscopic lymph node resection, the procedure consists of resection of the cervix, formation of an end-to-end anastomosis between the uterine corpus and vagina, and placement of a cerclage suture [54]. The postoperative MR appearance has been described, and reflects these anatomic changes [55]. In some cases, the appearance may mimic that of prior irradiation, resulting in a very small cervix, although in the case of trachelectomy, prominent suture susceptibility artifact may be seen (Fig. 16).

Summary

MR imaging has an established role in the investigation of the uterus and cervix. MR imaging is excellent for the staging of malignancy, although its exact clinical role has not been established universally.

References

[1] Nicolet V, Carignan L, Bourdon F, et al. MR imaging of cervical carcinoma: a practical staging approach. Radiographics 2000;20:1539–49.

[2] Kinkel K, Ariche M, Tardivon AA, et al. Differentiation between recurrent tumor and benign conditions after treatment of gynecologic pelvic carcinoma: value of dynamic contrast-enhanced subtraction MR imaging. Radiology 1997;204: 55–63.

[3] Brown MA, Mattrey RF, Stamato S, et al. MRI of the female pelvic using vaginal gel. AJR Am J Roentgenol 2005;185(5):1221–7.

[4] deSouza NM, Dina R, McIndoe GA, et al. Cervical cancer: value of an endovaginal coil magnetic resonance imaging technique in detecting small volume disease and assessing parametrial extension. Gynecol Oncol 2006;102(1):80–5.

[5] Amant F, Moerman P, Neven P, et al. Endometrial cancer. Lancet 2005;366(9484):491–505.

[6] Larson DM, Connor GP, Broste SK, et al. Prognostic significance of gross myometrial invasion with endometrial cancer. Obstet Gynecol 1996; 88:394–8.

[7] Kinkel K, Kaji Y, Yu KK, et al. Radiologic staging in patients with endometrial cancer: a meta-analysis. Radiology 1999;212:711–8.

[8] Frei KA, Kinkel K, Bonel HM, et al. Prediction of deep myometrial invasion in patients with endometrial cancer: clinical utility of contrast-enhanced MR imaging—a meta-analysis and Bayesian analysis. Radiology 2000;216:444–9.

[9] Sironi S, Colombo E, Villa G, et al. Myometrial invasion by endometrial carcinoma: assessment with plain and gadolinium-enhanced MR imaging. Radiology 1992;185:207–12.

[10] Liu PF, Krestin GP, Huch RA, et al. MRI of the uterus, uterine cervix, and vagina: diagnostic performance of dynamic contrast-enhanced fast multiplanar gradient-echo imaging in comparison with fast spin-echo T2-weighted pulse imaging. Eur Radiol 1998;8:1433–40.

[11] Frei KA, Kinkel K. Staging endometrial cancer: role of magnetic resonance imaging. J Magn Reson Imaging 2001;13:850–5.

[12] Kinkle K. Pitfalls in staging uterine neoplasm with imaging: a review. Abdom Imaging 2006;31:164–73.

[13] Tamai K, Togashi K, Ito T, et al. MR imaging findings of adenomyosis: correlation with histopathologic features and diagnostic pitfalls. Radiographics 2005;25:21–40.

[14] Seki H, Kimura M, Sakai K. Myometrial invasion of endometrial carcinoma: assessment with dynamic MR and contrast-enhanced T1-weighted images. Clin Radiol 1997;52:18–23.

[15] Matsushita H, Kodama S, Kase H, et al. [Usefulness of magnetic resonance imaging in the determination of cervical involvement in endometrial cancer]. Nippon Sanka Fujinka Gakkai Zasshi 1996;48:821–6 [in Japanese].

[16] Shibutani O, Joja I, Shiraiwa M, et al. Endometrial carcinoma: efficacy of thin-section oblique axial MR images for evaluating cervical invasion. Abdom Imaging 1999;24:520–6.

[17] Sato R, Jobo T, Kuramoto H. Parametrial spread is a prognostic factor in endometrial carcinoma. Eur J Gynaecol Oncol 2003;24:241–5.

[18] Tamussino KF, Reich O, Gucer F, et al. Parametrial spread in patients with endometrial carcinoma undergoing radical hysterectomy. Int J Gynecol Cancer 2000;10:313–7.

[19] Popovich MJ, Hricak H, Sugimura K, et al. The role of MR imaging in determining surgical eligibility for pelvic exenteration. AJR Am J Roentgenol 1993;160:525–31.

[20] Harisinghani MG, Saini S, Weissleder R, et al. MR lymphangiography using ultrasmall superparamagnetic iron oxide in patients with primary abdominal and pelvic malignancies: radiographic-pathologic correlation. AJR Am J Roentgenol 1999;172:1347–51.

[21] Acharya S, Hensley ML, Montag AC, et al. Rare uterine cancers. Lancet Oncol 2005;6(12):961–71.

[22] Ohguri T, Aoki T, Watanabe H, et al. MRI findings including gadolinium-enhanced dynamic studies of malignant, mixed mesodermal tumors of the uterus: differentiation from endometrial carcinomas. Eur Radiol 2002;12:2737–42.

[23] Rha SE, Byun JY, Jung SE, et al. CT and MRI of uterine sarcomas and their mimickers. AJR Am J Roentgenol 2003;181(5):1369–74.

[24] Lee HK, Kim SH, Cho JY, et al. Uterine adenofibroma and adenosarcoma: CT and MR findings. J Comput Assist Tomogr 1998;22(2):314–6.

[25] Tanaka YO, Nishida M, Tsunoda H, et al. Smooth muscle tumors of uncertain malignant potential and leiomyosarcomas of the uterus: MR findings. J Magn Reson Imaging 2004;20(6):998–1007.

[26] Metser U, Haider MA, Khalili K, et al. MR imaging findings and patterns of spread in secondary tumor involvement of the uterine body and cervix. AJR Am J Roentgenol 2003;180:765–9.

[27] Schiller JT, Lowy DR. Prospects for cervical cancer prevention by human papillomavirus vaccination. Cancer Res 2006;66(21):10229–32.

[28] American Joint Committee on Cancer: cancer staging manual. 6th edition. New York: Springer; 2002. p. 259–70.

[29] Holtz DO, Dunton C. Traditional management of invasive cervical cancer. Obstet Gynecol Clin North Am 2002;29:645–57.

[30] Covens A, Shaw P, Murphy J, et al. Is radical trachelectomy a safe alternative to radical hysterectomy for patients with stage IA-B carcinoma of the cervix? Cancer 1999;86:2273–9.

[31] Peppercorn PD, Jeyarajah AR, Woolas R, et al. Role of MR imaging in the selection of patients with early cervical carcinoma for fertility-preserving surgery: Initial experience. Radiology 1999;212:395–9.

[32] Morris M, Eifel PJ, Lu J, et al. Pelvic radiation with concurrent chemotherapy compared with pelvic and para-aortic radiation for high-risk cervical cancer. N Engl J Med 1999;340:1137–43.

[33] Subak LL, Hricak H, Powell CB, et al. Cervical carcinoma: computed tomography and magnetic resonance imaging for preoperative staging. Obstet Gynecol 1995;86:43–50.

[34] Bipat S, Glas AS, van der Velden J, et al. Computed tomography and magnetic resonance imaging in staging of uterine cervical carcinoma: a systematic review. Gynecol Oncol 2003;91:59–66.

[35] Hricak H, Powell CB, Yu KK, et al. Invasive cervical carcinoma: role of MR imaging in pretreatment work-up—cost minimization and diagnostic efficacy analysis. Radiology 1996;198:403–9.

[36] Shiraiwa M, Joja I, Asakawa T, et al. Cervical carcinoma: efficacy of thin-section oblique axial T2-weighted images for evaluating parametrial invasion. Abdom Imaging 1999;24:514–9.

[37] Hamm B, Kubik Huch RA, Fleige B. MR imaging and CT of the female pelvis: radiologic-pathologic correlation. Eur Radiol 1999;9:3–15.

[38] Hawighorst H, Knapstein PG, Weikel W, et al. Cervical carcinoma: comparison of standard and pharmacokinetic MR imaging. Radiology 1996;201:531–9.

[39] Semelka RC, Hricak H, Kim B, et al. Pelvic fistulas: appearances on MR images. Abdom Imaging 1997;22:91–5.

[40] Yang WT, Lam WW, Yu MY, et al. Comparison of dynamic helical CT and dynamic MR imaging in the evaluation of pelvic lymph nodes in cervical carcinoma. AJR Am J Roentgenol 2000;175: 759–66.

[41] Choi HJ, Kim SH, Seo SS, et al. MRI for pretreatment lymph node staging in uterine cervical cancer. AJR Am J Roentgenol 2006;187(5): W538–43.

[42] Follen M, Levenback CF, Iyer RB, et al. Imaging in cervical cancer. Cancer 2003;98:2028–38.

[43] Oguri H, Maeda N, Izumiya C, et al. MRI of endocervical glandular disorders: three cases of a deep nabothian cyst and three cases of a minimal-deviation adenocarcinoma. Magn Reson Imaging 2004;22:1333–7.

[44] Farley JH, Hickey KW, Carlson JW, et al. Adenosquamous histology predicts a poor outcome for patients with advanced-stage, but not early-stage, cervical carcinoma. Cancer 2003;97(9): 2196–202.

[45] Okamoto Y, Tanaka YO, Nishida M, et al. MR imaging of the uterine cervix: imaging-pathologic correlation. Radiographics 2003;23: 425–45.

[46] Okamoto Y, Tanaka YO, Nishida M, et al. Pelvic imaging: multicystic uterine cervical lesions. Can magnetic resonance imaging differentiate benignancy from malignancy? Acta Radiol 2004;45: 102–8.

[47] Ramos P, Ruiz A, Carabias E, et al. Mullerian adenosarcoma of the cervix with heterologous elements: report of a case and review of the literature. Gynecol Oncol 2002;84(1):161–6.

[48] Nguyen C, Montz FJ, Bristow RE. Management of stage I cervical cancer during pregnancy. Obstet Gynecol Surv 2000;55:633–43.

[49] Takushi M, Moromizato H, Sakumoto K, et al. Management of invasive carcinoma of the uterine cervix associated with pregnancy: outcome of intentional delay in treatment. Gynecol Oncol 2002;87(2):185–9.

[50] Fulcher AS, O'Sullivan SG, Segreti EM, et al. Recurrent cervical carcinoma: typical and atypical manifestations. Radiographics 1999;19:103–16.

[51] Manfredi R, Maresca G, Smaniotto D, et al. Cervical cancer response to neoadjuvant therapy: MR imaging assessment. Radiology 1998;209: 819–24.

[52] Scheidler J, Heuck AF, Steinborn M, et al. Parametrial invasion in cervical carcinoma: evaluation of detection at MR imaging with fat suppression. Radiology 1998;206:125–9.

[53] Yamashita Y, Harada M, Torashima M, et al. Dynamic MR imaging of recurrent postoperative cervical cancer. J Magn Reson Imaging 1996;6: 167–71.

[54] Hertel H, Kohler C, Grund D, et al. German Association of Gynecologic Oncologists (AGO). Radical vaginal trachelectomy (RVT) combined with laparoscopic pelvic lymphadenectomy: prospective multicenter study of 100 patients with early cervical cancer. Gynecol Oncol 2006; 103(2):506–11.

[55] Sahdev A, Jones J, Shepherd JH, et al. MR imaging appearances of the female pelvis after trachelectomy. Radiographics 2005;25(1):41–52.

ELSEVIER
SAUNDERS

MAGNETIC
RESONANCE
IMAGING CLINICS

Magn Reson Imaging Clin N Am 14 (2007) 471–487

MR Imaging Evaluation of the Adnexa

Claudia P. Huertas, MD[a,b], Michèle A. Brown, MD[c],
Richard C. Semelka, MD[a,*]

- MR imaging technique
- Normal anatomy
- Ovarian malignancies
  Epithelial origin
  Germ cell origin
  Sex cord–stromal origin

- *Secondary ovarian malignancy*
- Benign disease
  Nonneoplastic disease
  Benign ovarian neoplasms
- Summary
- References

MR imaging has become an important tool in the evaluation of patients with adnexal disease, and its role continues to evolve. Because of its multiplanar capability and superb soft tissue contrast, MR imaging provides localization and characterization of pelvic masses that often lead to specific diagnoses without the hazards of ionizing irradiation, which is particularly important in pregnant or adolescent women. Gadolinium-enhanced MR imaging provides the best assessment of complex adnexal masses to distinguish benign from malignant tumors, thus avoiding inappropriate management and reducing aggressive surgical intervention for benign diseases. In cases of malignant disease, MR imaging aids staging, surgical planning, and post-treatment surveillance [1–3].

MR imaging technique

Patients should fast for 4 to 6 hours and be asked to void immediately before scanning. A phased-array coil should be used routinely to improve signal-to-noise ratio [4,5]. Standard sequences include transverse T1-weighted spoiled gradient-echo, transverse T1-weighted gradient-echo with fat suppression, transverse echo-train spin-echo (ETSE) T2-weighted, sagittal or coronal breath-hold or single-shot ETSE (SS-ETSE), and postgadolinium gradient-echo with fat suppression. High-resolution ETSE T2-weighted sequences in the axial and sagittal planes can also be obtained. Sequential fast three-dimensional (3D) gradient-echo sequences are used for dynamic postgadolinium imaging.

Normal anatomy

Anatomically, the adnexa include the ovary, fallopian tube, round ligament, and structures arising from associated embryologic rests. The ovarian fossa is defined by the external iliac vessels anteriorly and by the ureter and internal iliac vessels posteriorly. In general, the ovaries are located lateral to

[a] Department of Radiology, University of North Carolina, 101 Manning Drive, CB7510, Chapel Hill, NC 27599-7510, USA
[b] Department of Radiology, Instituto Neurologico de Antioquia, Calle 55, 46-36, Medellin, Colombia
[c] Department of Radiology, University of California, San Diego Medical Center, 200 West Arbor Drive, San Diego, CA 92103-8756, USA
* Corresponding author.
E-mail address: richsem@med.unc.edu (R.C. Semelka).

the uterus and inferior to the fallopian tubes, although there is some variability in their position. Ovarian size varies with age; in the neonate, the volume of the ovaries is approximately 1 cm³, increasing in size after 6 years of age; in premenarchal girls, ovarian volumes range from 2 to 4 cm³ [6], and in premenopausal women, ovarian volumes range from 5 to 8 cm³. A decrease in size begins at the age of 30 years, with more pronounced atrophy after menopause. Histologically, the ovary is divided into the medullary (central) region containing stromal cells, lymphatics, blood vessels, and nerves and the cortical (peripheral) region containing follicles in differing stages of maturation. The ovaries are supplied from the ovarian artery and the ovarian branch of the uterine artery. Venous drainage differs between the left and right, with the left ovarian vein draining into the left renal vein and the right ovarian vein draining directly into the inferior vena cava (IVC). The lymphatic drainage of the ovaries follows the venous drainage into para-aortic nodes.

In patients of reproductive age, normal ovaries can usually be identified in MR images. In postmenopausal women, ovaries are not consistently seen in up to 60% of patients. On T1-weighted images, the signal intensity of the ovary is similar to that of the myometrium. If present, follicles are typically hyperintense on T2-weighted images, and their identification is useful to help differentiate the ovary from adjacent small bowel and vessels (Fig. 1). After administration of gadolinium, ovarian enhancement varies, reflecting the hormonal status. In premenopausal women, ovarian enhancement tends to be less than that of the myometrium, whereas in postmenopausal women, enhancement is equivalent [7,8]. The fallopian tubes are encased within the superior portion of the broad ligament. The normal tube is approximately 10 cm in length and has a 1- to 4-mm luminal diameter [9]. The normal fallopian tube is not routinely seen on MR imaging.

Ovarian malignancies

Ovarian cancer is the second most common gynecologic malignancy, but it has the highest mortality rate of all gynecologic malignancies, with an overall 5-year survival rate of 46% [10]. The main reason for this poor prognosis is advanced stage at the time of diagnosis (Fig. 2). Ovarian cancer is a "silent" disease, with the preclinical phase estimated to be less than 2 years, and most of these cancers develop de novo [11]. Screening efforts have neither been successful nor cost-effective even in high-risk patients. Cancer antigen 125 (CA-125) is a useful marker, especially in postmenopausal women but has false-positive elevations in premenopausal patients, pregnancy, endometriosis, leiomyoma, and pelvic inflammatory disease [11]. Ovarian cancer is primarily a diagnosis of middle-aged and older women. Risk factors include early menarche, low parity, older age at first pregnancy, late menopause, and hereditary syndromes (eg, familial site-specific ovarian cancer syndrome, breast ovarian cancer syndrome, Lynch syndrome). Ultrasound (US) is the primary imaging modality for detection and characterization of adnexal masses; however, as many as 20% of adnexal lesions in premenopausal women are classified as indeterminate by US [12]. Contrast-enhanced MR imaging has been reported to have as high as 91% to 95% overall accuracy for differentiating benign from malignant tumors [12,13]. Improved pretreatment characterization helps to guide appropriate treatment in each patient. Although MR imaging cannot differentiate histologically different subtypes of tumors, there are some specific findings that are more characteristic of particular lesions. Several criteria suggestive of malignancy have been described, including size (>4–6 cm, depending on the series), wall thickening (>3 mm), multiple (>5) septa (>3 mm thick), and the presence of bilateral masses; however, the MR imaging findings most predictive of malignancy are solid to cystic lesions, the presence of vegetations in a cystic lesion, and necrosis in a solid lesion [12]. Ancillary findings include ascites, peritoneal implants, and lymphadenopathy. In up to 80% of cases, the CA-125 level is elevated at presentation and the level can be followed to assess for response to treatment. A normal value does not exclude the presence of tumor, however. Potential problems in lesion detection with MR imaging include small (<2 cm) lesion size and occasional difficulty in determining whether a large adnexal mass is unilateral or bilateral [12].

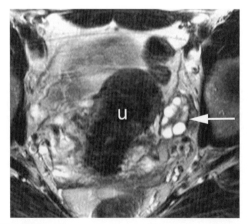

Fig. 1. Normal ovary. Transverse T2-weighted ETSE image demonstrates a normal left ovary with multiple follicles (*arrow*) adjacent to the uterus (u).

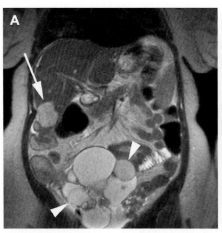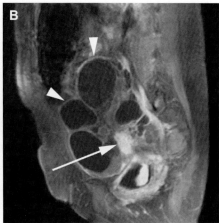

Fig. 2. Disseminated ovarian mucinous cystadenocarcinoma. Coronal T2-weighted SS-ETSE (*A*) and sagittal gadolinium-enhanced, fat-suppressed, T1-weighted gradient-echo (*B*) images demonstrate a complex septated cystic lesion arising from the pelvis (*arrowheads*). Note the capsular cystic liver metastasis in the inferior right lobe (*arrow, A*). There is enhancement of the septations and solid component of the mass (*arrow, B*). The peritoneum was also seen to enhance.

Malignant neoplasms nearly always require laparotomy. A staging laparotomy consists of a total abdominal hysterectomy, bilateral salpingo-oophorectomy, infracolic omentectomy, biopsies from multiple random peritoneal sites, and pelvic and para-aortic lymphadenectomy. Stages are assigned according to the International Federation of Gynecology and Obstetrics (FIGO) schema. CT imaging is frequently used for preoperative staging assessment of ovarian cancer, with a reported sensitivity of 63% to 79% and a specificity of 100%. Sensitivity is decreased for peritoneal implants less than 1 cm in size [14]. MR imaging is similar in accuracy to CT in regard to local staging and may be a more accurate modality for detecting peritoneal metastasis outside the true pelvis, with reported advantages of depiction of disease involving the peritoneum, omentum, bowel, osseous vascular structures, and perihepatic implants [15]. Prognosis depends on tumor stage, residual disease after initial surgery (tumor <1.5 cm), and tumor grade. MR imaging determination of malignant disease extent assists treatment planning in surgical candidates or can identify nonresectable disease [16]. After surgery and chemotherapy, MR imaging may also be helpful to detect residual or recurrent disease even in a subclinical stage [17], and it has been comparable to laparotomy reassessment and superior to serum CA-125 values alone in patients with treated ovarian cancer (**Fig. 3**) [18].

Ovarian tumors are classified on the basis of cell origin as epithelial tumors, germ cell tumors, sex cord–stromal cell tumors, and metastatic tumors (**Box 1**).

Epithelial origin

Surface epithelial tumors are by far the most common type of malignant ovarian tumor, accounting for more than 85% of the cases. Malignant subtypes include serous, mucinous, clear cell, endometrioid, and undifferentiated cancers [19]. Approximately 75% to 85% of patients with epithelial neoplasms present with peritoneal disease, and even women with apparently localized disease may have metastases detected in peritoneal washings or biopsies outside the pelvis [19]. Tumor may also spread to the para-aortic and pelvic lymph nodes. Another category includes those tumors that have borderline features or low malignant potential. These tumors have an excellent prognosis despite sharing histologic features of frankly malignant masses; the quality they lack is destructive growth without stromal invasion [19].

Serous

Cancers arising from the serous cell type account for half of all ovarian malignancies [20], with bilateral disease in 50% of the patients. Serous cancers are predominantly unilocular cysts. As the degree of cellular differentiation decreases, the incidence of hemorrhage, solid elements, and necrosis increases. On MR imaging, papillary projections, seen as intermediate-signal-intensity projections within a cystic lesion that enhance with gadolinium, are important hallmarks to indicate tumors of serous origin (**Fig. 4**) [20], and this finding is highly suggestive of borderline or malignant tumors [19]; however, they can also be present in some benign serous cystadenomas. Approximately 30% contain

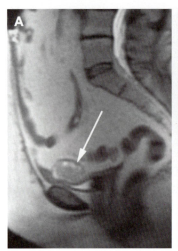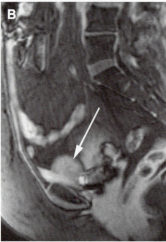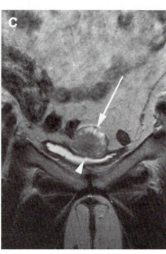

Fig. 3. Recurrent mixed epithelial ovarian cancer. Sagittal T2-weighted SS-ETSE (*A*); sagittal gadolinium-enhanced, fat-suppressed, T1-weighted gradient-echo (*B*); and coronal 512 high-resolution T2-weighted ETSE (*C*) images in a patient with previous resection of ovarian carcinoma show recurrent disease superior to the bladder (*arrow*) with serosal invasion demonstrated by loss of the normal hypointensity in the bladder wall (*arrowhead, C*).

calcifications as psammoma bodies [20], which are not well seen on MR imaging.

Mucinous

Mucinous cancers are less common and account for 10% of malignant ovarian tumors [14]. These lesions are larger, frequently multilocular, and more often unilateral compared with serous tumors. On MR imaging, they appear as a multiloculated lesion with septations of variable thickness that enhance with gadolinium and display a "stained glass" appearance derived from proteinaceous or mucinous content causing different signal intensities on T1- and T2-weighted images within each locule

(Fig. 5) [21]. Areas of hemorrhage, necrosis, and solid elements may be seen.

Endometrioid

Cancers of the endometrioid cell type represent 15% of ovarian cancers. Bilateral involvement is seen in 30% to 50%. They may arise within the ovary or within foci of endometriosis, and endometrioid cancers are the most common neoplasm associated with endometriosis, followed by clear cell carcinoma [22]. They are almost always malignant and are associated with endometrial hyperplasia or endometrial carcinoma in up to 30% of cases. Imaging features are nonspecific, with lesions generally composed of a mixture of cystic and solid elements with papillary projections seen uncommonly. Rarely, the tumor may appear as a purely

---

Box 1:   Malignant ovarian tumors

Epithelial tumors (85%)
- Serous (50%)
- Mucinous (10%)
- Endometrioid (15%)
- Clear cell (5%)
- Undifferentiated
- Borderline (15%)

Germ cell tumors (~5%)
- Dysgerminoma
- Endodermal sinus tumor
- Embryonal cell carcinoma
- Immature teratoma
- Choriocarcinoma

Sex cord–stromal tumors (~5%)
- Granulosa cell tumor
- Other tumors

Metastatic tumors (5%–10%)

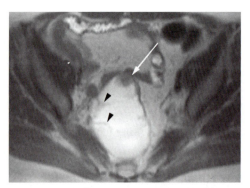

Fig. 4. Serous papillary ovarian carcinoma. Transverse T2-weighted image demonstrates a unilocular predominantly cystic lesion with irregular septa (*arrowheads*) and a peripheral solid nodule (*arrow*).

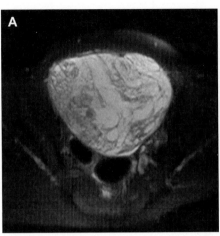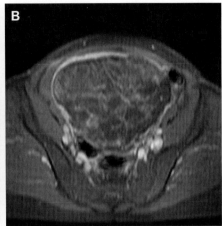

Fig. 5. Mucinous cystadenocarcinoma. Axial fat-suppressed T2-weighted SS-ETSE (*A*) and gadolinium-enhanced, fat-suppressed, T1-weighted gradient-echo (*B*) images show a large multilobulated mass with enhancing septa.

solid lesion. The diagnosis should also be considered when an enhancing nodule is seen within a predominantly cystic endometrioma.

Clear cell

Cancers arising from the clear cell type are less common, comprising 5% of ovarian cancers, and are bilateral in approximately 13% of cases. Clear cell tumors are always malignant; however, unlike the other cell types, at least three quarters of them present with local disease (stage I) and carry a better prognosis. These are generally unilocular cystic tumors with solid mural nodules, which may be few in number and mimic serous tumors. The presence of proteinaceous material or hemorrhage may alter T1- and T2-weighted signal intensities [23]. Similar to endometrioid cancers, these lesions may arise in endometriomas (Fig. 6). In the case of a hemorrhagic mass, it may be difficult to detect nodule enhancement and subtraction images may be useful in this setting.

Undifferentiated

These include tumors that do not fit into any of the four cell types of origin described previously. Undifferentiated epithelial cancers carry the poorest prognosis, with widespread disease generally present at diagnosis.

Borderline tumor

These tumors are a distinct histologic and clinical disease; they are diagnosed in up to 15% of patients, usually younger women, and exhibit a better prognosis compared with serous tumors [24]. These tumors demonstrate a greater proliferation of papillary projections than benign cystadenomas and fewer solid components than cystadenocarcinomas.

No imaging feature allows confident differentiation from other epithelial carcinomas, however [25].

Germ cell origin

Malignant germ cell tumors account for less than 5% of ovarian cancers. Among ovarian tumors identified in female patients younger than 21 years of age, 60% belong to this group but only 30% are malignant. Many of these are associated with serum marker levels.

Dysgerminoma

This tumor is the ovarian counterpart of seminoma of the testis [26] and represents the most common malignant germ cell tumor in young women. Usually, the prognosis is excellent. Serum lactate dehydrogenase (LDH) is elevated in up to 95% of patients [11]. Dysgerminoma presents as a solid multilobulated tumor with prominent fibrovascular septa. Calcification may be present in a speckled pattern. In contrast to yolk sac tumors, foci of hemorrhage or necrosis are rare, allowing some differentiation between these tumors [27].

Endodermal sinus tumor

Also known as a yolk sac tumor, an endodermal sinus tumor is the second most common malignant germ cell cancer and usually occurs in the second decade of life. In most patients, α-fetoprotein is prominently elevated and is used to monitor treatment outcome. The tumor grows rapidly and has a poor prognosis. The MR imaging appearance has been described as a large solid mass with internal cysts, almost always associated with necrosis or hemorrhage, and with greater enhancement than the uterus [28].

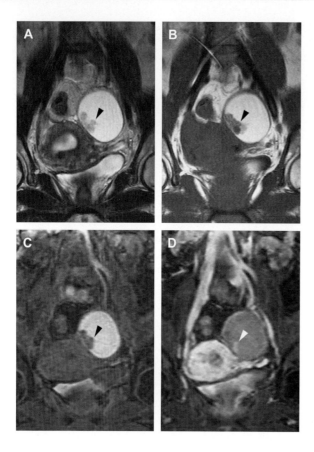

Fig. 6. Clear cell carcinoma arising in an endometrioma. Coronal T2-weighted ETSE (*A*); T1-weighted gradient-echo (*B*); and fat-suppressed T1-weighted gradient-echo images before (*C*) and after (*D*) administration of gadolinium show a hemorrhagic left ovarian mass with a small solid component that enhances (*arrowhead*). Enhancement is often difficult to detect in hemorrhagic lesions, and subtraction images may be helpful.

Immature teratoma

These rare germ cell tumors comprise 1% of this group. They usually arise during the first 2 decades of life. The tumor contains immature tissue from all three germ cell layers. These tumors are frequently unilateral, grow rapidly, and are composed of a prominent solid component with scattered calcifications and small foci of fat (Fig. 7). The tumor

capsule is not always identified and is usually perforated, because these tumors tend to spread by seeding the peritoneum [29].

Sex cord–stromal origin

These tumors arise from stromal cells (fibroblasts, theca cells, and Leydig cells) and primitive sex cords (granulosa cells) in the ovary. Sex cord–stromal

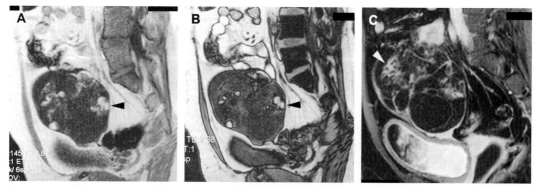

Fig. 7. Immature teratoma. Sagittal T1-weighted gradient-echo images obtained in-phase (*A*), out-of-phase (*B*), and with fat suppression after gadolinium administration (*C*) show a large ovarian mass containing small amounts of fat (*arrowheads; A, B*) as well as signal intensities consistent with fluid and soft tissue. The soft tissue attenuation areas enhance after gadolinium administration (*arrow, C*).

tumors affect all age groups but account for less than 5% of all malignant ovarian tumors. Most of them are hormonally active, exhibiting mainly estrogenic effects.

Granulosa cell tumor

Granulosa cell tumors are divided in two types, adult and juvenile; both excrete estrogen. Adult granulosa tumors are more common than the juvenile type and occur in postmenopausal women. Presentation may be with abnormal uterine bleeding, because these tumors are associated with endometrial hyperplasia, polyps, and cancer in 3% to 35% of the cases [30]. The histologic pattern and gross appearance are variable, ranging from a predominantly solid to a uni- or multilocular cystic mass [30]. On MR imaging, the typical appearance is a solid lesion, with variable amounts of cystic and fibrotic changes and intratumoral hemorrhage. These tumors are of intermediate signal intensity on T1-weighted images and heterogeneously high signal intensity on T2-weighted images. After administration of gadolinium, solid areas enhance but areas of cystic change or hemorrhage do not. In contrast to epithelial tumors, granulosa cell tumors are confined to the ovary in most patients and do not tend to seed the peritoneum. Also well demonstrated on MR images are the associated uterine changes attributable to estrogenic influence, including uterine enlargement and thickening of the endometrium [31]. Because of early presentation, surgery is often curative; however, they have been reported to recur even 10 to 20 years after diagnosis.

Secondary ovarian malignancy

Metastases

Functioning highly vascularized ovaries of premenopausal women are more receptive to secondary involvement than ovaries in postmenopausal women. The mode of spread of metastatic disease can be by direct extension from adjacent organs, hematogenous, lymphatic, or serosal implantation of cells shed into the peritoneal cavity [32]. Ovarian metastasis can be divided into two groups: Krukenberg tumors (30%–40%) and others. The term *Krukenberg tumor* specifically refers to tumors in which malignant mucin-filled signet ring cells are found within the ovarian stroma. At least 80% result from gastric carcinoma, but tumors arising from the breast, colon, and appendix, and, less commonly, from the gallbladder, pancreas, biliary tract, urinary bladder, and cervix can also give rise to these histologic features [32]. Krukenberg tumors are frequently bilateral and generally have cystic

and solid components; the cystic components are variable in signal on T1- and T2-weighted images, largely reflecting the content of mucin or blood [33]. Solid components show variable enhancement after administration of gadolinium, which may be intense [33,34]. The MR imaging appearance of metastatic disease to the ovary is influenced by the primary malignancy and route of spread. For example, metastasis from colon cancer frequently presents as a multiloculated unilateral cystic lesion resembling a primary ovarian tumor [32].

Lymphoma

Most ovarian involvement with lymphoma is part of disseminated disease. The most common forms are non-Hodgkin lymphoma in children and younger women and large cell lymphoma in adults. The diagnosis may be suspected based on the clinical setting. On MR imaging, ovarian lymphoma generally appears as bilateral masses with homogeneous hypointensity on T1-weighted images and slight hyperintensity on T2-weighted images without necrosis, hemorrhage, or calcification. Contrast enhancement is mild to moderate and is more conspicuous with fat suppression techniques [35]. Physiologic follicles may be preserved [36].

Benign disease

Nonneoplastic disease

Functional ovarian cysts

The diagnosis of uncomplicated functional cysts is generally straightforward. When complicated by hemorrhage, differentiation from endometriomas and neoplasms may be difficult. Resolution of a cyst on follow-up imaging classifies it as functional. Absence of papillary projections is an important feature that allows differentiation from neoplastic cysts. Endometriomas generally have high signal intensity on T1-weighted images and T2 shortening ("shading") [37], which is a typical feature of endometrioma and is unusual in corpus luteal cysts. Endometriosis is commonly multifocal, and implants are often seen in the cul-de-sac. In the absence of multiplicity or T2 shading, the distinction from a hemorrhagic cyst is sometimes difficult and follow-up imaging may be helpful.

Theca-lutein cysts

Elevated circulating levels of human chorionic gonadotropin (b-HCG), usually seen in women with gestational trophoblastic disease (46%) or ovarian hyperstimulation syndrome for infertility, can cause gross enlargement of the ovaries, generally between 6 and 12 cm, even up to 20 cm, because of the presence of multiple, bilateral, and often multilocular theca-lutein cysts, which measure up to 4 cm. They are usually asymptomatic and commonly disappear 2 to 4 months after resolution of the condition; however, women may sometimes present in pain if a cyst undergoes rupture or hemorrhage or if the ovary torses. On MR imaging, theca-lutein cysts have a variable appearance with low to high signal on T1-weighted images and high signal on T2-weighted images (Fig. 8) [38,39]. If there is an associated hypervascular endometrial mass, gestational trophoblastic disease should be considered.

Paraovarian and peritoneal cysts

Paraovarian cysts may account for 10% to 20% of adnexal masses and represent benign or malignant cysts that can arise within the broad ligament or parovarium [40]. Often, these represent hydatid cysts of Morgagni that arise from Müllerian duct remnants and are frequently localized at the fimbriated end of the fallopian tube. Paraovarian cysts are generally asymptomatic, although large cysts may undergo torsion or develop hemorrhage and cause pelvic pain. On MR imaging, uncomplicated cysts have signal characteristics of simple fluid. Paraovarian cysts are round or ovoid and are sometimes multiple or bilateral, and they may be indistinguishable from ovarian cysts unless a normal ipsilateral ovary is identified separately from the cystic lesion. Peritoneal inclusion cysts or peritoneal pseudocysts are collections of ovulatory ovarian fluid, usually around the ovary, that lack a true wall and require two conditions for formation: an ipsilateral functioning ovary and adhesions in which the fluid is trapped. Usually, there is a history of prior abdominopelvic surgery or endometriosis; they tend to conform to surrounding structures and are often triangular or irregular in shape rather than round. These distinguishing morphologic features are well shown by MR imaging [41]. The

diagnosis should be suspected when a normal ovary or ovarian tissue is seen within the wall of the pseudocyst (Fig. 9). If left untreated, they tend to grow because of continued accumulation of fluid [42].

Polycystic ovaries

Polycystic ovarian syndrome (PCOS) represents a spectrum of disease caused by a hormone imbalance; it leads to stimulation of the ovaries without maturation of a dominant follicle, which results in chronic anovulation. On MR images, polycystic ovaries are normal to large in size with multiple small peripheral follicles of uniform size that are consistently bright on T2-weighted images and dark on T1-weighted images. A dark capsule and prominent central stroma can be seen on T2-weighted images (Fig. 10) [43,44]. Ovarian volume is normal in 30% of the patients, and overlap exists between the MR imaging appearance of normal and polycystic ovaries [44]. Patients are typically treated for the presenting complaints of infertility, menstrual irregularity, or androgen excess. Because of the unopposed estrogen seen in anovulation, patients with PCOS are at increased risk for endometrial cancer [45].

Endometriosis

Endometriosis is a common and usually benign entity that affects women in their reproductive years, with a prevalence of approximately 10% in the general population. It is defined as the presence of endometrial epithelium and stroma outside the uterine cavity [47]. In order of decreasing frequency, the most common sites of involvement are the ovaries, uterine ligaments, cul-de-sac, serosal uterine surface, fallopian tubes, rectosigmoid, and bladder dome [47,48]. Other potential sites of involvement are the distal ureters, and rare distant

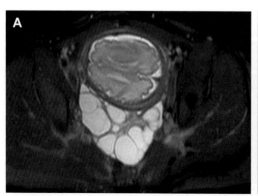
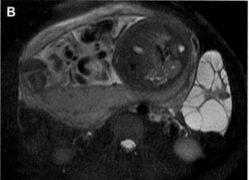

Fig. 8. Theca-lutein cysts in a pregnant patient. Axial fat-suppressed T2-weighted SS-ETSE images in a pregnant woman show multiple large simple cysts with enlargement of the right (*A*) and the left (*B*) ovaries.

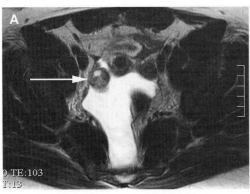
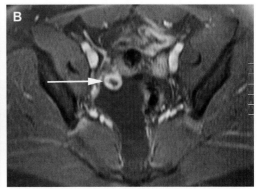

Fig. 9. Peritoneal inclusion cyst. Axial T2-weighted ETSE (*A*) and fat-suppressed, postgadolinium, T1-weighted gradient-echo (*B*) images show a large fluid collection that conforms to surrounding structures such as bowel. At the periphery of the collection, ovarian tissue is seen containing an enhancing corpus luteum cyst (*arrow*).

foci may arise in a variety of location, such as the pleural surface. Endometriosis is a complex and probably multifactorial disorder with three main postulated causes: metastatic, metaplastic, and induction of cells [46]. Malignant transformation occurs in less than 1% of cases, most commonly to endometrioid carcinoma and clear cell carcinoma. Laparoscopy is the standard of reference for the diagnosis and staging of endometriosis, although pitfalls exist, including atypical lesions or those obscured by dense adhesions [48]. In such cases, MR imaging has a potential role in the diagnosis. On MR imaging, endometriomas appear as single or multiple thick-walled cystic lesions, with surrounding fibrosis and adhesions to adjacent structures caused by inflammatory reaction.

Endometriomas are typically hyperintense on T1-weighted images, and small lesions are best demonstrated with fat suppression (Fig. 11) [49]. Lesions are typically of low signal intensity on T2-weighted images (shading). The sensitivity of MR imaging for detecting endometriomas ranges from 90% to 92%, and the specificity ranges from 91% to 98% [50]. The diagnosis of small endometrial implants is more elusive. Endometriosis implants may enhance with gadolinium, and this finding may raise suspicion of malignancy. MR imaging may not detect extremely small superficial lesions that can be seen at laparoscopy; however, MR imaging may surpass laparoscopy at detecting deep pelvic endometriosis, which is more frequently symptomatic [51]. Endometriosis may also occur in extrapelvic locations, most commonly the abdominal wall in patients with a history of cesarean section, and abdominal wall endometriomas may be entirely solid (Fig. 12) [52].

Ovarian torsion

Torsion of the ovary occurs most frequently in children and adolescents and is secondary to ovarian masses in most cases but can occur in normal ovaries, especially in children and pregnant women (Fig. 13). Although most patients present with acute onset of pelvic pain, some patients complain of episodic pain, presumably related to intermittent ovarian torsion. In the earliest stages, only the venous flow is restricted, with resulting congestion, edema, and interstitial hemorrhage causing enlargement of the ovary. If left untreated, the arterial flow is progressively restricted with hemorrhagic necrosis of the ovary and any associated mass. Pathologic and radiologic changes reflect the degree of vascular compromise. MR imaging shows an enlarged edematous ovary with peripheral follicles. Complete absence of enhancement indicates

Fig. 10. Polycystic ovaries. Coronal 512 high-resolution T2-weighted ETSE image shows both ovaries with multiple tiny peripheral follicles and low signal intensity in the medullary stroma.

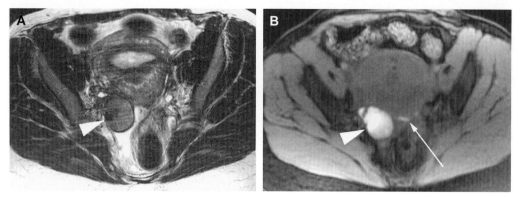

Fig. 11. Endometriosis. Axial T2-weighted ETSE (*A*) and T1-weighted fat-suppressed gradient-echo (*B*) images show an endometrioma in the right side (*arrowhead*) with low signal intensity in the T2-weighted image and high signal intensity in the T1-weighted fat-suppressed image reflecting blood, with smaller implants in the cul-de-sac demonstrated in the T1-weighted fat-suppressed image (*arrow, B*).

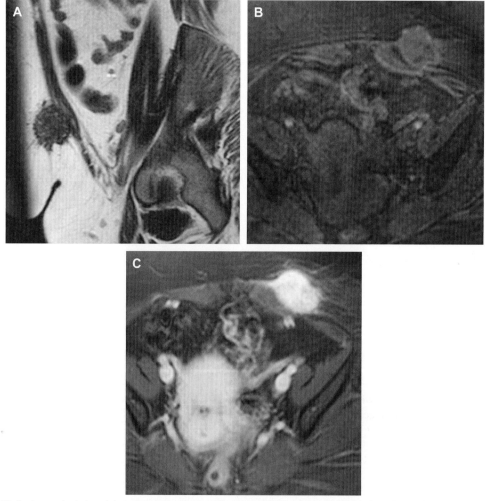

Fig. 12. Endometriosis involving the abdominal wall. Sagittal T2-weighted ETSE (*A*) and axial fat-suppressed T1-weighted gradient-echo images before (*B*) and after (*C*) administration of gadolinium show a spiculated mass in the left anterior abdominal wall that is hypointense on T2-weighted images, isointense on T1-weighted images, and enhances intensely with gadolinium.

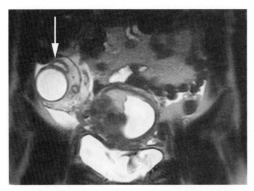

Fig. 13. Ovarian torsion. Coronal T2-weighted SS-ETSE image in a pregnant woman with right lower quadrant pain shows an enlarged edematous right ovary (*arrow*) with a cyst and adjacent fluid. Ovarian torsion was confirmed at surgery.

significant arterial compromise; however, if there is only venous congestion, some enhancement is present, and this feature may be better seen with the use of MR subtraction imaging [53]. Additional but nonspecific findings include uterine deviation toward the torsed ovary, tube thickening, ascites, and hemorrhage within the lesion, with a high signal intensity rim surrounding the adnexal mass on T1-weighted images [54]. MR imaging findings of massive ovarian edema (up to 40 cm) with increased signal intensity on T2-weighted images, sometimes with multiple peripheral follicles, have also been described when there is twisting of the vascular pedicle without hemorrhagic infarction and there is no underlying mass [55].

Pelvic inflammatory disease and tubo-ovarian abscess

Pelvic inflammatory disease (PID) is common in women of reproductive age and refers to a variety of pelvic infections. Patients usually present with fever, pelvic pain, cervical motion tenderness, and a vaginal discharge accompanied by an elevated blood level of C-reactive protein. Noncomplicated PID and tubo-ovarian abscess (TOA) are commonly diagnosed on the basis of clinical findings and US. Approximately 20% of women may be afebrile, however, with nonspecific symptoms, inconclusive US findings, or chronic stages, and to distinguish TOA from malignancy, MR imaging evaluation may be helpful. MR imaging in PID depicts the extent of inflammation because of ill-defined hyperintensity on fat-suppressed T2-weighted images that enhances markedly on postgadolinium, fat-suppressed, T1-weighted images [56]. These areas are shown as hypointense curvilinear stranding on routine T1-weighted imaging. Pyosalpinx is seen as a fluid-filled tube with purulent material, which

has variable signal intensity on T1- and T2-weighted images, with the fluid-debris level associated with thick walls that enhance on postcontrast images. TOA may appear as a tubular, thick-walled, fluid-filled mass with a hypointense center on T1-weighted images and hyperintense or heterogeneous on T2-weighted images, with intense wall enhancement [57,58]. MR imaging is also helpful in detecting other potential causes of symptoms, such as endometrioma, ovarian neoplasm, infected ovarian cyst, and abscess from another source (eg, Crohn disease, appendicitis, diverticulitis).

Hydrosalpinx

Occlusion of the fimbriated end of the tube produces tubal dilation resulting in a hydrosalpinx. If complicated by hemorrhage or infection, the term *hematosalpinx* or *pyosalpinx* is used, respectively. The causes of the occlusion include PID, endometriosis, adjacent tumors, and adhesions from prior surgery. On MR images, hydrosalpinx appears as a tubular fluid-filled structure folded on itself to form an S or C shape [59]. It is well demonstrated using multiplanar imaging revealing a multicystic structure corresponding to the dilated tube (Fig. 14), at times showing the cause of the obstruction.

Ectopic pregnancy

Most extrauterine pregnancies are located in the fallopian tubes, followed by the ovaries. The incidence of ectopic pregnancy is increasing principally because of the use of ovulation-stimulating drugs [60]. Most ectopic pregnancies are suspected on a clinical and hormonal basis and are confirmed

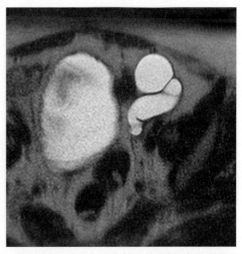

Fig. 14. Hydrosalpinx. Axial T2-weighted SS-ESTE image demonstrates a tubular fluid-filled structure in the left adnexa.

with transvaginal US. A potential advantage of MR imaging is its ability to localize the implantation site of a cornual or cervical ectopic pregnancy precisely, which is important for proper management. MR imaging features of the entity include hematosalpinx, enhancement of the fallopian tube wall, a gestational sac-like structure, bloody ascites, and a heterogeneous adnexal mass. The hematoma and the ascites show increased signal intensity on fat-suppressed T1-weighted images [61]. An enhancing tree-like region within a heterogeneous mass has been reported to represent villus-containing fibrin strands in the fetoplacental tissue, and this finding, only demonstrated with MR imaging, is especially useful to identify unusual locations of an ectopic pregnancy [62].

Benign ovarian neoplasms

As with their malignant counterparts, benign ovarian neoplasms are classified according to cell type (Box 2).

Epithelial origin
Benign epithelial tumors include serous, mucinous, and transitional cell (Brenner tumors). Most are cystadenomas, usually serous or mucinous. Although each one has characteristic MR imaging features, overlap exists. Differentiation is not of paramount importance, because treatment is identical. Serous cystadenomas are common and usually present as a thin-walled unilocular cyst, although they may be multilocular. Although papillary projections may occur in benign epithelial tumors, this finding should raise suspicion of malignancy [63]. In general, benign epithelial

Box 2: Benign ovarian tumors

Epithelial tumors
- Serous (25%)
- Mucinous (20%)
- Brenner (2%–3%)
- Cystadenofibromas and adenofibromas

Germ cell tumors
- Mature teratomas (20%–50%)
- Monodermal teratomas (3%)

Sex cord–stromal tumors
- Fibrothecoma (20%)
- Sclerosing stromal tumor

tumors have fewer and smaller projections than borderline or frankly malignant tumors [25].

Mucinous cystadenomas are usually multilocular and lack papillary projections, facilitating differentiation from serous lesions, and they also tend to be larger than serous cystadenomas. On MR imaging, mucinous cystadenomas usually demonstrate multiple locules with different signal intensity on T1- and T2-weighted images because of their mucin or protein content (Fig. 15) [63]. Mucinous cystadenomas may also be unilocular or have few septa, resembling serous cystadenoma.

Brenner tumors, also called transitional cell tumors, arise from the surface epithelium of the ovary and contain nests of urothelium-like cells and dense stroma [64]. Most are benign and account for 2% to 3% of all ovarian neoplasms. Brenner tumors are usually small (<2 cm), but they are associated with other ovarian tumors in approximately 30% of cases, usually in the ipsilateral ovary. These

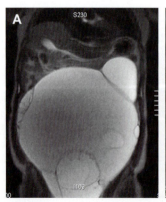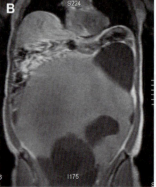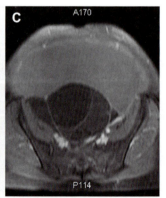

Fig. 15. Mucinous cystadenoma. Coronal T2-weighted SS-ESTE (*A*); coronal T1-weighted gradient-echo (*B*); and axial gadolinium-enhanced, fat-suppressed, T1-weighted gradient-echo (*C*) images show a large cystic mass originating in the pelvis and extending into the upper abdomen with septa and different signal intensities within the locules. There is subtle contrast enhancement of the septa but no evident papillary projections. MR imaging cannot reliably distinguish between borderline and malignant tumor based in imaging features.

tumors have signal characteristics similar to fibromas, with decreased homogeneous signal intensity on T2-weighted images because of the dense fibrous stroma, which is sometimes associated with amorphous calcification [24,65], and larger tumors may show cystic areas [64]. Cystadenofibromas are cystic epithelial neoplasms in which fibrous stroma is a major component in addition to epithelial cells. Adenofibromas contain even more fibrous components. These tumors are usually benign. The MR imaging appearance is variable and depends on the amount of solid tissue that appears as extremely low signal on T2-weighted images [66]. Cystadenofibromas may also appear nearly entirely cystic on MR images, mimicking cystadenomas, or may have thick septa and solid nodules, mimicking malignant tumors (Fig. 16) [67]. The septations and solid component may be extremely dark on T2-weighted images, reflecting their fibrous nature.

Germ cell origin

Mature cystic teratoma or dermoid cyst is the only benign tumor of germ cell origin and is the most common ovarian neoplasm [68]. These tumors are composed of variable amounts of mature endodermal (mucinous or ciliated epithelium), mesodermal (muscle or fat), and ectodermal (brain or skin) elements [29]. Management consists of conservative surgery depending on the size of the tumor and the desire to preserve fertility. Mature teratomas show variability in their appearance, ranging from mainly cystic or fatty masses to mixed lesions, based on the expression of the germ cell layers [68]. The characteristic MR imaging feature is fat, which is present in approximately 95% of mature cystic teratomas. The fat within the lesion has signal characteristics of gross fat signal on all sequences (Fig. 17). T1-weighted images combined with out-of-phase imaging or chemically selective

fat suppression improve diagnostic confidence, with accuracy up to 96% [69]. Out-of-phase imaging has a particular advantage in lesions with only small amounts of fat. Other findings include fluid-fluid levels, layering debris, low signal intensity calcification (usually teeth), and Rokitansky nodules (dermoid plugs attached to the cyst wall) [1,29,70]. Monodermal teratomas are a subset of teratomas that are composed predominantly or uniquely of one tissue type, such as struma ovarii, struma carcinoid, and tumors with neural differentiation. Struma ovarii account for 3% of all mature teratomas and are composed of mature thyroid tissue. MR imaging findings may be more characteristic than US findings and demonstrate a complex multilocular mass with variable signal intensity because of the differences in viscosity within the locules, associated with solid components, which demonstrate substantial enhancement after administration of gadolinium and correspond to thyroid tissue (Fig. 18). No fat is identified within these tumors [29,71].

Sex chord–stromal origin

Fibroma, thecoma, and fibrothecoma arise from the stromal elements of the ovary and are forms of a spectrum composed of fibrous cells, thecal cells, or a combination of the two, sometimes with overlap in the histologic appearance. Tumors that contain thecal cells are associated with increased estrogen, and 15% of the patients have concomitant endometrial hyperplasia or frank endometrial carcinoma in 29% of the cases. In fact, many of these tumors are discovered during evaluation of abnormal bleeding. The MR imaging characteristics for all these tumors are similar: hypointensity on T1- and T2-weighted images. After administration of gadolinium, these tumors have variable enhancement, with reports of negligible

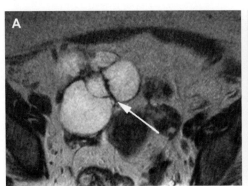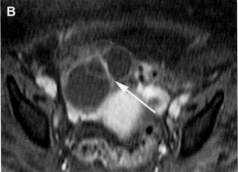

Fig. 16. Benign cystadenofibroma. Axial T2-weighted ETSE (*A*) and gadolinium-enhanced, fat-suppressed, T1-weighted gradient-echo (*B*) images show a complex multiseptated mass arising from the right ovary with thick irregular septa that are dark on T2-weighted images (*arrow, A*) and enhance with gadolinium (*arrow, B*).

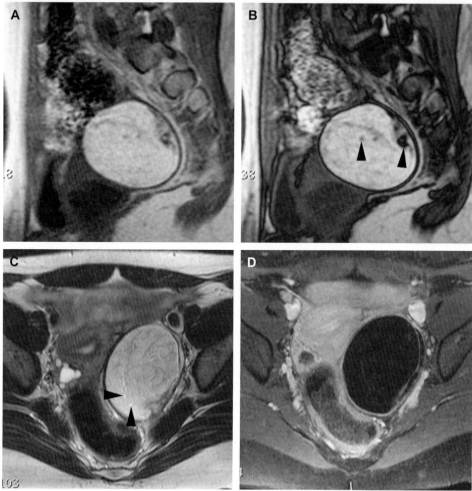

Fig. 17. Dermoid cyst. Sagittal T1-weighted gradient-echo images obtained in-phase (*A*) and out-of-phase (*B*); axial T2-weighted ETSE image (*C*); and fat-suppressed, postgadolinium, T1-weighted gradient-echo (*D*) image show a left ovarian mass consisting almost entirely of fat. Small internal foci cause chemical shift artifact of the second kind with signal loss on out-of-phase images (*arrowheads, B*) and chemical shift artifact of the first kind attributable to spatial misregistration (*arrowheads, C*). There is no significant enhancement within the cyst after administration of gadolinium.

and avid enhancement. Atypical high T2 signal attributable to pronounced microscopic myxomatous change has been also reported [30,72–74]. Sometimes, there is difficulty in differentiating exophytic leiomyomas from fibrous ovarian tumors because of the similar signal characteristics; in these cases, it is useful to identify the "bridging vascular sign," which describes curvilinear tortuous vascular structures crossing between the uterus and the pelvic mass [75]. Detection of compressed ovarian tissue surrounding an ovarian tumor is also useful.

Sclerosing stromal tumor of the ovary is a rare benign lesion that presents in women younger than 30 years of age and is generally associated with complaints of menstrual irregularity. MR imaging

findings include a large mass with a pattern described as pseudolobular, composed of hyperintense cystic components and variable amount of fibrous stroma, reflecting the histopathologic features of the tumor [76]. These tumors are highly vascular with intense early contrast enhancement that progresses in a centripetal fashion [24,30,77]. Resection is curative.

Summary

MR imaging is a robust and reproducible evaluation that has inherent high tissue contrast and multiplanar image capabilities not available in other modalities. The recent technical developments of fast

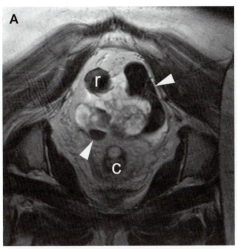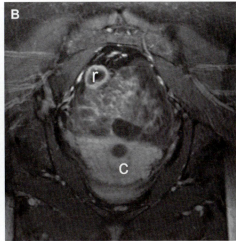

Fig. 18. Struma ovarii. Angled axial T2-weighted ETSE (*A*) and fat-suppressed, postgadolinium, T1-weighted gradient-echo (*B*) images demonstrate a multilocular mass between the rectum (r) and cervix (c), which contains a nabothian cyst. There is variable signal intensity within locules, including regions of extremely dark signal on T2-weighted images (*arrowheads, A*), and no gross fat in the lesion. Portions of the mass enhance intensely with contrast, corresponding to thyroid tissue.

imaging sequences and parallel imaging techniques minimize artifacts and provide superior imaging quality. In women of childbearing age and pregnant women, the lack of ionizing radiation and safety of gadolinium are of paramount importance. Some benign entities can be diagnosed by MR imaging with a high degree of confidence, such as teratomas, endometriomas, simple and hemorrhagic cysts, fibromas, and hydrosalpinx. In the case of malignant lesions, MR imaging may improve lesion characterization, staging, and follow-up.

References

[1] Jeong YY, Outwater EK, Kang HK. Imaging evaluation of ovarian masses. Radiographics 2000;20: 1445–70.

[2] Thurnher S, Hodler J, Baer S, et al. Gadolinium-DOTA enhanced MR imaging of the adnexal tumors. J Comput Assist Tomogr 1990;14:939–49.

[3] Stevens SK, Hricak H, Stern JL. Ovarian lesions: detection and characterization with gadolinium enhanced MR imaging at 1.5 T. Radiology 1991; 181:481–8.

[4] Smith RC, Reinhold C, McCauley TR, et al. Multicoil high resolution fast spin-echo MR imaging of the female pelvis. Radiology 1992;184:671–5.

[5] Hayes CE, Dietz MJ, King BF, et al. Pelvic imaging with phased array coils: quantitative assessment of signal-to-noise ratio improvement. J Magn Reson Imaging 1992;2:321–6.

[6] Garel L, Dubois J, Grignon A, et al. US of the pediatric female pelvis: a clinical perspective. Radiographics 2001;21(6):1393–407.

[7] Outwater EK, Talerman A, Dunton C. Normal adnexa uteri specimens: anatomic basis of MR imaging features. Radiology 1996;201:751–5.

[8] Dooms GC, Hricak H, Tscholakoff D. Adnexal structures: MR imaging. Radiology 1986;58: 639–46.

[9] Rowling SE, Ramchandani P. Imaging of the fallopian tubes. Semin Roentgenol 1996;31: 299–311.

[10] American Cancer Society. Cancer facts and figures: 1998. Atlanta (GA): American Cancer Society; 1998. p. 13.

[11] Togashi K. Ovarian cancer: the clinical role of US, CT and MRI. Eur Radiol 2003;13:87–104.

[12] Hricak H, Chen M, Coakley FV, et al. Complex adnexal masses: detection and characterization with MR imaging multivariate analysis. Radiology 2000;214:39–46.

[13] Sohaib SAA, Sahdev A, Van Trappen P, et al. Characterization of adnexal lesions on MR imaging. AJR Am J Roentgenol 2003;180: 1297–304.

[14] Funt S, Hricak H. Ovarian malignancies. Top Magn Reson Imaging 2003;14(4):329–38.

[15] Low RN, Semelka RC, Worawattanakul S, et al. Extrahepatic abdominal imaging in patients with malignancy: comparison of MR imaging and helical CT with subsequent surgical correlation. Radiology 1999;210:625–32.

[16] Asher SM, Takahama J, Jha RC. Staging of gynecologic malignancies. Top Magn Reson Imaging 2001;12(2):105–29.

[17] Low RN, Saleh F, Song SYT, et al. Treated ovarian cancer: comparison of MR imaging with serum CA-125 level and physical examination—a longitudinal study. Radiology 1999;211:519–28.

[18] Low RN, Duggan B, Barone R, et al. Treated ovarian cancer: MR imaging, laparotomy reassessment, and serum CA-125 values compared with clinical outcome at 1 year. Radiology 2005; 235:918–26.

[19] Ozols RF, Rubin SC, Thomas GM, et al. Epithelial ovarian cancer. In: Hoskins WJ, Perez CA, Young RC, editors. Principles and practice of gynecologic oncology. Philadelphia: Lippincott; 2000. p. 981–1058.

[20] Sutton CL, McKinney CD, Jones JE, et al. Ovarian masses revisited: radiologic and pathologic correlation. Radiographics 1992;12:853–77.

[21] Tanaka YO, Nishida M, Kurosaki Y, et al. Differential diagnosis of gynaecological "stained glass" tumors on MRI. Br J Radiol 1999;72:414–20.

[22] Tanaka YO, Yoshizako T, Nishida M, et al. Ovarian carcinoma in patients with endometriosis: MR imaging findings. AJR Am J Roentgenol 2000;175:1423–30.

[23] Matsuoka Y, Ohtomo K, Araki T, et al. MR imaging of clear cell carcinoma of the ovary. Eur Radiol 2001;11:946–51.

[24] Jung SE, Lee JM, Rha SE, et al. CT and MR imaging of ovarian tumors with emphasis on differential diagnosis. Radiographics 2002;22(6): 1305–25.

[25] deSouza NM, O'Neill R, McIndoe GA, et al. Borderline tumors of the ovary: CT and MRI features and tumor markers in differentiation from stage I disease. AJR Am J Roentgenol 2005;184(3): 999–1003.

[26] Brammer HM III, Buck JL, Hayes WS, et al. Malignant germ cell tumors of the ovary: radiologic-pathologic correlation. Radiographics 1990,10: 715–24.

[27] Tanaka YO, Kurosaki Y, Nishida M, et al. Ovarian dysgerminoma: MR and CT appearance. J Comput Assist Tomogr 1994;18:443–8.

[28] Yamaoka T, Togashi K, Koyama T, et al. Yolk tumor of the ovary: radiologic-pathologic correlation in four cases. J Comput Assist Tomogr 2000;24:605–9.

[29] Outwater EK, Siegelman ES, Hunt JL. Ovarian teratomas: tumor types and imaging characteristics. Radiographics 2001;21:475–90.

[30] Jung SE, Rha SE, Lee JM, et al. CT and MRI findings of sex cord-stromal tumor of the ovary. AJR Am J Roentgenol 2005;185:207–15.

[31] Tanaka YO, Tsunoda H, Kitagawa Y, et al. Functioning ovarian tumors: direct and indirect findings at MR imaging. Radiographics 2004; 24(Suppl 1):S147–66.

[32] Young RH, Scully RE. Metastatic tumors in the ovary. In: Blaustein A, editor. Pathology of the female genital tract. New York: Springer-Verlag; 1994. p. 939–74.

[33] Kim SH, Kim WH, Park KJ, et al. CT and MR findings of Krukenberg tumors. Comparison with primary ovarian tumors. J Comput Assist Tomogr 1996;20:393–8.

[34] Ha HK, Baek SY, Kim SH, et al. Krukenberg's tumor of the ovary: MR imaging features. AJR Am J Roentgenol 1995;164:1435–9.

[35] Ferrozzi F, Tognini G, Bova D, et al. Non-Hodgkin lymphomas of the ovaries: MR findings. J Comput Assist Tomogr 2000;24:416–20.

[36] Mitsumori A, Joja I. MRI appearance of non-Hodgkin's lymphoma of the ovary. AJR Am J Roentgenol 1999;173:245.

[37] Outwater EK, Schiebler ML, Owens RS, et al. MRI characterization of hemorrhagic adnexal masses: a blinded reader study. Radiology 1993;186: 489–94.

[38] Hricak H, Demas BE, Braga CA, et al. Gestational trophoblastic neoplasm of the uterus: MR assessment. Radiology 1986;161:11–6.

[39] Barton JW, McCarthy SM, Kohorn EI, et al. Pelvic MR imaging findings in gestational trophoblastic disease, incomplete abortion, and ectopic pregnancy: are they specific? Radiology 1993; 186:163–8.

[40] Kier R. Nonovarian gynecologic cysts: MR imaging findings. AJR Am J Roentgenol 1992;158: 1265–9.

[41] Kurachi H, Murakami T, Nakamura H, et al. Imaging of peritoneal pseudocysts: value of MR imaging compared with sonography and CT. AJR Am J Roentgenol 1993;160:589–91.

[42] Jain KA. Imaging of peritoneal inclusion cysts. AJR Am J Roentgenol 2000;174:1559–63.

[43] Outwater EK, Schiebler ML. Magnetic resonance imaging of the ovary. Radiol Clin North Am 1994;2:245–74.

[44] Kimura I, Togashi K, Kawakami S, et al. Polycystic ovaries: implications of diagnosis with MR imaging. Radiology 1996;201:549–52.

[45] Guzick DS. Polycystic ovary syndrome. Obstet Gynecol 2004;103:181–93.

[46] Woodward PJ, Sohaey R, Mezzetti TP Jr. Endometriosis: radiologic-pathologic correlation. Radiographics 2001;21:193–216.

[47] Clement PB. Pathology of endometriosis. Pathol Annu 1990;3:234–55.

[48] Bis KG, Vrachliotis TG, Agrawal R, et al. Pelvic endometriosis: MR imaging spectrum with laparoscopic correlation and diagnostic pitfalls. Radiographics 1997;17:639–55.

[49] Ha HK, Lim YT, Kim HS, et al. Diagnosis of pelvic endometriosis: fat suppressed T1-weighted vs. conventional MR images. AJR Am J Roentgenol 1994;163:127–31.

[50] Togashi K, Nishimura K, Kimura I, et al. Endometrial cyst: diagnosis with MR imaging. Radiology 1991;180:73–8.

[51] Bazot M, Darai E, Hourani R, et al. Deep pelvic endometriosis: MR imaging for diagnosis and prediction of extension of disease. Radiology 2004;232:379–89.

[52] Hensen JH, Van Breda Vriesman AC, Puylaert JB. Abdominal wall endometriosis: clinical presentation and imaging features with emphasis on

sonography. AJR Am J Roentgenol 2006;186(3): 616–20.

[53] Kimura I, Togashi K, Kawakami S, et al. Ovarian torsion: CT and MR imaging appearances. Radiology 1994;190:337–41.

[54] Rha SE, Byun JY, Jung SE, et al. CT and MR imaging features of adnexal torsion. Radiographics 2002;22:283–94.

[55] Lee AR, Kim KH, Lee BH, et al. Massive edema of the ovary: imaging findings. AJR Am J Roentgenol 1993;161:343–4.

[56] Dohke M, Watanabe Y, Okumura A, et al. Comprehensive MR imaging of acute gynecologic diseases. Radiographics 2000;20:1551–66.

[57] Tukeva TA, Aronen HJ, Karjalainen PT, et al. MR imaging in pelvic inflammatory disease: comparison with laparoscopy and US. Radiology 1999; 210:209–16.

[58] Ha HK, Lim GY, Cha ES, et al. MR imaging of tubo-ovarian abscess. Acta Radiol 1995;36: 510–4.

[59] Outwater EK, Siegelman ES, Chiowanich P, et al. Dilated fallopian tubes: MR imaging characteristics. Radiology 1998;208:463–9.

[60] Brown M, Ascher SM, Semelka RC. Adexa. In: Semelka RC, editor. Abdominal-pelvic MRI. 2nd edition. Hoboken (NJ): John-Wiley & Sons, Inc.; 2006. p. 1333–82.

[61] Kataoka ML, Togashi K, Kobayashi H, et al. Evaluation of ectopic pregnancy by magnetic resonance imaging. Hum Reprod 1999;14: 2644–50.

[62] Ha HK, Jung JK, Kang SK, et al. MR imaging in the diagnosis of rare forms of ectopic pregnancy. AJR Am J Roentgenol 1993;160:1229–32.

[63] Ghossain MA, Buy JN, Ligneres C, et al. Epithelial tumors of the ovary: comparison of MR and CT findings. Radiology 1991;181:863–70.

[64] Moon WJ, Koh BH, Kim SK, et al. Brenner tumor of the ovary: CT and MR findings. J Comput Assist Tomogr 2000;24:72–6.

[65] Outwater EK, Siegelman ES, Kim B, et al. Ovarian Brenner tumors: MR imaging characteristics. Magn Reson Imaging 1998;16:1147–53.

[66] Outwater EK, Siegelman ES, Talerman A, et al. Ovarian fibromas and cystadenofibromas: MRI of the fibrous component. J Magn Reson Imaging 1997;7:465–71.

[67] Cho SM, Byun JY, Rha SE, et al. CT and MRI findings of cystadenofibromas of the ovary. Eur Radiol 2004;14:798–804.

[68] Rha SU, Byun JY, Jung SE, et al. Atypical CT and MRI manifestations of mature ovarian cystic teratomas. AJR Am J Roentgenol 2004;183:743–50.

[69] Stevens SK, Hricak H, Campos Z. Teratomas versus cystic hemorrhagic adnexal lesions: differentiation with proton-selection fat saturation MR imaging. Radiology 1993;186:481–8.

[70] Togashi K, Nishimura K, Itoh K, et al. Ovarian cystic teratomas: MR imaging. Radiology 1987; 162:669–73.

[71] Matsuki M, Kaji Y, Matsuo M, et al. Struma ovarii: MRI findings. Br J Radiol 2000;73:87–90.

[72] Schwartz RK, Levine D, Hatabu H, et al. Ovarian fibroma: findings by contrast-enhanced MRI. Abdom Imaging 1997;22:535–7.

[73] Troiano RN, Lazzarini KM, Scoutt LM, et al. Fibroma and fibrothecoma of the ovary: MR imaging findings. Radiology 1997;204:795–8.

[74] Ueda J, Furukawa T, Higashino K, et al. Ovarian fibroma of high signal intensity on T2-weighted MR image. Abdom Imaging 1998;23:657–8.

[75] Kim JC, Kim SS, Park YJ. "Bridging vascular sign" in the MR diagnosis of exophytic uterine leiomyoma. J Comput Assist Tomogr 2000;24:57–60.

[76] Ihara N, Togashi K, Todo G, et al. Sclerosing stromal tumor of the ovary: MRI. J Comput Assist Tomogr 1999;23:555–7.

[77] Torricelli P, Caruso Lombardi A, Boselli F, et al. Sclerosing stromal tumor of the ovary: US, CT, and MRI findings. Abdom Imaging 2002;27: 588–91.

MAGNETIC
RESONANCE
IMAGING CLINICS

Magn Reson Imaging Clin N Am 14 (2007) 489–501

ELSEVIER
SAUNDERS

MR Imaging Evaluation of Acute Abdominal Pain During Pregnancy

Aytekin Oto, MD

- Technique and safety
- Clinical indications
  Gastrointestinal system
  Biliary system

Urinary system
Gynecologic indications
- Summary
- References

Acute abdominal pain in the pregnant patient presents unique diagnostic and therapeutic challenges. The clinical evaluation of pregnant patients is confounded by physiologic and anatomic changes related to pregnancy [1,2]. The gravid uterus displaces the bowel, causes compression of the ureters, and limits the physical examination. The appendix demonstrates a progressive upward displacement during the course of the pregnancy, altering the typical clinical presentation of acute appendicitis [3]. Mild leukocytosis, anemia, and elevated alkaline phosphatase are considered normal during pregnancy. Because clinical and laboratory findings cannot reliably suggest an etiology, diagnostic imaging is often required in the evaluation of pregnant women presenting with an acute abdomen.

Ultrasound (US) is a safe imaging modality for pregnant patients and is accurate in evaluation of the ovaries, gravid uterus, fetus, kidneys, and gallbladder [4,5]. It is operator dependent, however, and factors like a gravid uterus and bowel gas may limit the evaluation of the entire abdomen. CT is an excellent method to evaluate the acute abdomen but is of limited use in pregnant patients because of the exposure of the fetus to a considerable radiation dose and iodinated contrast material. The International Commission on Radiological Protection

recently recommended that if the expected dose for the fetus is high, one should question whether the diagnosis could be obtained without using ionizing radiation [6].

MR imaging can provide a systematic cross-sectional evaluation of the entire abdomen with excellent anatomic resolution and without exposing the fetus to ionizing radiation. MR imaging is often used in the obstetric setting as a problem-solving tool for maternal and fetal diseases and has been shown to be useful for the evaluation of various causes of acute abdominal pain [7–9]. Recently, studies describing MR imaging evaluation of acute abdominal pain during pregnancy have increased in number, reflecting the increased use of MR imaging in this challenging clinical setting [10–13]. The purpose of this review is to describe the MR imaging technique and findings of various abnormalities causing acute abdominal pain in pregnant patients.

Technique and safety

Pregnant patients are informed about MR imaging safety issues, and informed consent is obtained before each study. Our current MR imaging protocol does not require any specific patient preparation. Some investigators recommend administration of negative oral contrast 1 hour before the

Department of Radiology, University of Texas Medical Branch at Galveston, 301 University Boulevard, Galveston, TX 77550–0709, USA
E-mail address: ayoto@utmb.edu

1064-9689/07/$ – see front matter © 2007 Elsevier Inc. All rights reserved.
mri.theclinics.com

doi:10.1016/j.mric.2007.01.003

examination to provide filling of the cecum and better identification of bowel segments [9]. A phased-array coil provides a superior signal-to-noise ratio, but in larger patients and toward the end of pregnancy, a body coil may be necessary. If patients feel uncomfortable lying supine in the scanner (especially in the third trimester), imaging can be obtained with the patient in the lateral decubitus position, decreasing the pressure on the inferior vena cava [8].

T2-weighted imaging in three orthogonal planes with single-shot fast spin echo (SSFSE) or half-Fourier acquisition single-shot spin echo (HASTE) sequences (repetition time [TR] = infinite, echo time [TE] = 90 milliseconds) forms the backbone of the MR imaging protocol. The field of view is typically 35 cm, and the matrix size is 160 to 192 × 256 (phase, frequency encoding). An additional T2-weighted sequence with fat saturation (SSFSE/HASTE or fast spin echo [FSE]) is performed to improve the detection of inflammation or characterization of fatty adnexal lesions. An axial T1-weighted image is also included in the protocol. This image can be a breath-hold spoiled gradient echo or a respiratory gated FSE sequence. The resolution of T1-weighted FSE is superior to that of the gradient echo version and can be helpful for detection of small structures, such as a normal appendix.

On review of the noncontrast images, the radiologist may consider the administration of intravenous contrast in selected cases. If postcontrast imaging is needed, two-dimensional (2D) or three-dimensional (3D) gradient-recalled echo (GRE) T1-weighted images can be acquired after administration of gadolinium at a dose of 0.1 mmol/kg.

In addition to these routine sequences, axial 2D time-of-flight images (TR/TE of 25 milliseconds/minimum) can be obtained from the renal veins to the symphysis pubis to screen for a venous clot [9]. If magnetic resonance cholangiopancreatography (MRCP) or magnetic resonance urography is indicated, a thin-slice, 3D, heavily T2-weighted FSE sequence can be performed. Steady-state free-precession sequences (fast imaging employing steady-state acquisition [FIESTA], true fast imaging with steady-state precession [FISP], balanced fast field echo [FFE]) can provide motion-free images of the abdomen, nicely depicting the outline of the bowel segments and vessels. Monitoring of the MR imaging examination by a radiologist is recommended to customize the studies individually and to limit the scan time to a minimum while answering the clinical question.

There are no reported deleterious effects, but the safety of MR imaging with respect to the fetus has not been definitively established. In 1991, the Safety Committee of the Society for Magnetic Resonance Imaging stated that "MR imaging may be used in pregnant women if other non-ionizing forms of diagnostic imaging are inadequate or if the examination provides important information that would otherwise require exposure to ionizing radiation" [14]. MR imaging uses the static, time-varying, and radiofrequency electromagnetic fields, and all these fields can potentially cause adverse effects on the fetus. Animal studies on the safety of fetal MR imaging are not conclusive and are sometimes conflicting [15]. A small number of studies in human fetuses using regular MR imaging protocols have not revealed any harmful effects on the fetus, however [16–19]. Because of a lack of conclusive data, MR imaging of pregnant women should be used when the benefits outweigh the theoretic risks, and extra caution should be exercised in the first trimester [20].

Gadolinium-based contrast agents cross the placenta and have been shown to increase skeletal malformations in animal studies [8]. There are no human data obtained from long-term controlled studies, but it is suggested that gadolinium-based agents be used only in the second and third trimesters when the benefits outweigh the risks [8].

Clinical indications

Gastrointestinal system

Acute appendicitis

Acute appendicitis is the most common cause of acute abdomen in pregnancy, occurring in approximately 1 in 1500 deliveries [2]. In 1923, Baer and colleagues [21] described the cephalad migration of the appendix based on barium enema findings in pregnant patients, and these results were also recently confirmed by MR imaging [3]. Because of this upward migration, the localization of pain is not as specific as in nonpregnant patients for diagnosis of acute appendicitis. It is also important to realize that there is a physiologic increase in the white blood cell count in pregnancy. These difficulties can lead to a delay in diagnosis that can be associated with serious complications. The incidence of fetal loss increases from 3% to 5% without rupture to 30% with ruptured appendicitis [2]. There is a need for an accurate and safe noninvasive imaging tool to evaluate pregnant patients with acute appendicitis.

MR imaging can show an enlarged appendix with a thick wall and associated periappendiceal inflammation or abscess in patients with acute appendicitis (Fig. 1) [10–13]. Incesu and colleagues [22] reported that an inflamed appendix demonstrates marked wall enhancement with slight distention. In a series of pediatric patients, accurate diagnosis of acute appendicitis could be made even without administration of intravenous

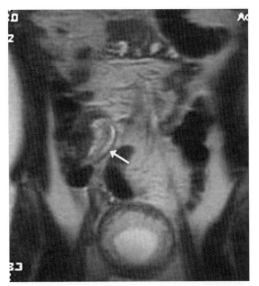

Fig. 1. Acute appendicitis. Coronal T2-weighted SSFSE image shows a dilated thick-walled appendix (*arrow*) extending medially from the cecum.

contrast material [23]. Several articles from different centers investigating the role of MR imaging for evaluation of acute appendicitis specifically in pregnant patients have been published in recent years [10–13]. In their small series of 12 patients, Cobben and colleagues [10] concluded that MR imaging may be a good alternative to CT in pregnant patients with indeterminate sonographic findings. The two other series with relatively larger study populations (n = 23 and n = 29) showed that MR imaging allows diagnosis of acute appendicitis and other causes of right-sided abdominal pain, such as ovarian torsion, pelvic abscesses, ureteral stones, or biliary obstruction, by providing a systematic evaluation of abdominal and pelvic organs [11,12]. In another series of 50

patients, the overall sensitivity, specificity, and accuracy of MR imaging in diagnosis of acute appendicitis were reported as 100%, 93.6%, and 94%, respectively [13]. Intravenous contrast was not administered to most patients included in these series.

MR imaging can also show the normal appendix, helping to exclude the diagnosis of acute appendicitis and saving pregnant patients from unnecessary appendectomies. More than 40% of patients who undergo appendectomy in the second and third trimesters have a normal appendix, and preterm contractions are common in as many as 83% of pregnant patients who undergo appendectomy [24]. MR imaging can be an excellent modality in pregnant women who present with acute abdominal pain and in whom a normal appendix is not visualized at US [13].

Bowel obstruction

Small bowel obstruction is the second most common nonobstetric indication for surgical intervention during pregnancy, occurring in approximately 1 of 3000 deliveries [1,2]. The cause is adhesions in 60% to 70% of cases, and it is more common in first pregnancies and during the first trimester or postpartum period [2]. The second most common cause of bowel obstruction in pregnancy is volvulus, which is present in approximately 25% of the cases [25]. Small bowel obstruction is associated with significant fetal morbidity and mortality, and its incidence has been climbing because of an increase in the number of abdominal operations performed.

MR imaging, particularly using single-shot echo train spin echo sequences, allows evaluation of the entire gastrointestinal tract and can show the presence and level of small bowel obstruction with a high degree of accuracy (**Figs. 2 and 3**) [26].

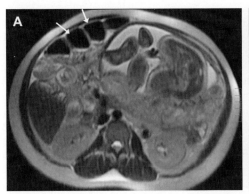
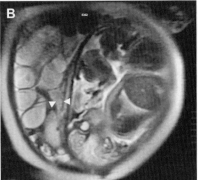

Fig. 2. Small bowel obstruction. (*A*) Axial T2-weighted SSFSE image shows dilated small bowel (*arrows*). (*B*) Coronal T2-weighted SSFSE image shows dilated and normal-caliber small bowel (*arrowheads*) in the right lower quadrant. Surgery confirmed small bowel obstruction at the ileum attributable to adhesions (*Courtesy of* Michèle A. Brown, MD, San Diego, CA).

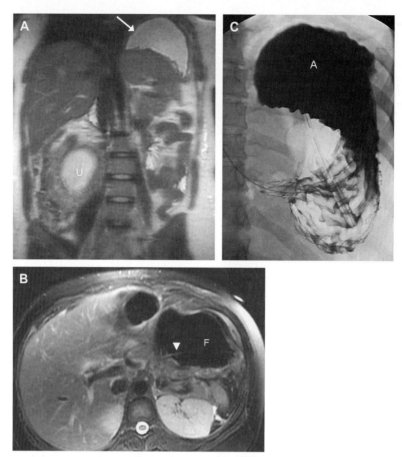

Fig. 3. Gastric volvulus. (*A*) Coronal T2-weighted SSFSE image shows a cystic structure (*arrow*) representing the dilated gastric antrum in the left subdiaphragmatic space. The gravid uterus is seen in the abdomen (u). (*B*) Axial T2-weighted fat-saturated FSE image shows that the fundus (F) and cardia of the stomach are inferior to their expected anatomic location, suggestive of gastric volvulus. A nasogastric tube (*arrowhead*) allows confident identification of the esophagogastric junction. (*C*) Upper gastrointestinal study confirms the mesenteroaxial volvulus by demonstrating the superior position of the antrum (A) compared with the fundus. Subsequent emergency surgery was performed.

Inflammatory bowel disease

Inflammatory bowel disease (IBD) peaks in incidence during a woman's reproductive years and can present with diarrhea, abdominal pain, fever, and anorectal disease. IBD activity is mostly independent of pregnancy, but there are reports stating that one third of women with IBD relapse during pregnancy [27,28]. Differentiating the signs and symptoms of IBD from physiologic changes related to pregnancy or other obstetric, gynecologic, or surgical conditions may be difficult [29].

Such imaging techniques as upper gastrointestinal studies, barium enemas, small bowel follow-through, enteroclysis, and CT are commonly used to establish a diagnosis; to assess the location, extent, and severity of disease; and to detect the complications of IBD. MR imaging has intrinsic advantages over these techniques, including noninvasiveness and the absence of ionizing radiation. The lack of artifacts from magnetic susceptibility and peristalsis makes the SSFSE sequences ideal for bowel imaging. An inflamed bowel wall demonstrates increased signal on T2-weighted images, especially at the acute phase (Fig. 4) [30,31]. Maccioni and colleagues [32] also demonstrated a correlation between biologic activity and wall signal intensity on T2-weighted images. Another sequence suitable for evaluation of IBD without intravenous contrast is T2/T1-weighted steady-state acquisition (FIESTA or true FISP). In addition to evaluating the bowel lumen and the wall, MR imaging can accurately diagnose extraluminal complications, such as intestinal obstruction, fistula, or abscess formation (Fig. 5) [30]. MR imaging can facilitate the planning of interventional treatment by providing thorough cross-sectional imaging of an abscess.

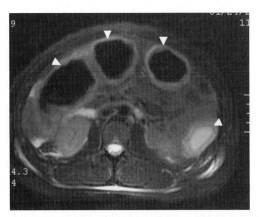

Fig. 4. Acute colitis. Axial T2-weighted fat-saturated FSE image shows increased signal and thickening of the transverse and descending colon wall (*arrowheads*) in this pregnant patient with history of IBD.

Biliary system

Acute cholecystitis

Pregnancy increases bile lithogenicity and sludge formation as a consequence of increased cholesterol synthesis by estrogen and impaired gallbladder motility by progesterone [33]. Acute cholecystitis is the third most common nonobstetric surgical emergency during pregnancy. The incidence is 1 to 8 per 10,000 pregnancies [1]. Cholecystectomy is best performed in the second trimester because it is associated with miscarriage during the first trimester and with premature labor during the third trimester [34].

US is the initial imaging study for diagnosis of cholelithiasis and cholecystitis. MR imaging can also demonstrate gallbladder wall thickening, a distended gallbladder with gallstones, and increased pericholecystic signal on T2-weighted images, however (Fig. 6) [35]. Regan and colleagues [36] reported that MR imaging with single-shot turbo

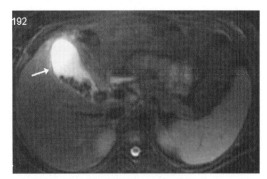

Fig. 6. Acute cholecystitis. Axial T2-weighted fat-saturated FSE image shows multiple stones in a distended gallbladder with a thickened wall (*arrow*).

spin echo is an ideal imaging modality in the initial evaluation of acute biliary pain and is comparable to US in the preoperative evaluation of acute cholecystitis.

Biliary obstruction

Symptomatic choledocholithiasis is not common during pregnancy. US can demonstrate the gallstones and dilatation of the biliary system, but its sensitivity in detection of choledocholithiasis is low. When biliary obstruction is clinically suspected, MRCP can display the biliary anatomy and detect small stones in the common bile duct with a high sensitivity and specificity (Fig. 7) [37]. MRCP using respiratory-triggered, 3D, fast-recovery fast spin echo sequences provides better image quality and better visualization of the biliary tree [38]. MRCP can also save patients from unnecessary endoscopic retrograde cholangiopancreatography (ERCP) by demonstrating a normal common bile duct. Rare causes for biliary obstruction, such as Mirizzi syndrome, choledochal cysts, or

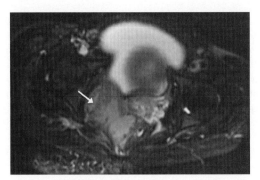

Fig. 5. Perirectal abscess. Axial T2-weighted fat-saturated FSE image reveals a thick-walled collection (*arrow*) in the right perirectal space. The patient had history of Crohn's disease, and the abscess was percutaneously drained.

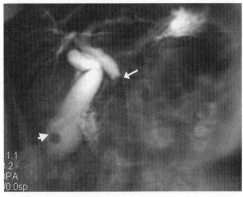

Fig. 7. Choledocholithiasis. Stone (*arrow*) in the distal common bile duct causing biliary obstruction is seen on the coronal thick-slab MRCP image. Note an additional stone in the gallbladder (*arrowhead*).

intrahepatic biliary stones, can also be successfully diagnosed using high-resolution MRCP sequences (Fig. 8) [39].

Acute pancreatitis

Acute pancreatitis complicates approximately 1 of every 3300 pregnancies, most commonly occurring during the third trimester and postpartum [40]. The etiology is gallstones in most cases. Pregnancy does not significantly alter the clinical or laboratory presentation of the disease. Serum amylase and lipase levels remain reliable markers of acute pancreatitis during pregnancy. US is used to detect cholelithiasis and bile duct dilatation but cannot optimally evaluate the distal common bile duct and pancreas. MR imaging can have an important role in staging the severity of acute pancreatitis and imaging its complications, such as pseudocysts [41]. T1-weighted GRE images with fat suppression before and after intravenous contrast are the most important sequences for pancreatic evaluation. T2-weighted SSFSE images allow evaluation of the biliary and pancreatic ducts and accurate depiction of peripancreatic inflammation, pseudocysts, and fluid collections without administration of intravenous gadolinium (Fig. 9) [41].

Urinary system

Mild hydronephrosis or hydroureter is common during pregnancy because of compression of the ureter by the gravid uterus and decreased muscle tone of the urinary tract from elevated progesterone levels [1]. This physiologic hydronephrosis is more

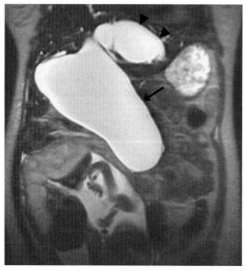

Fig. 8. Choledochal cyst. Coronal T2-weighted SSFSE image shows a severely dilated common bile duct (*arrow*) and intrahepatic biliary tree (*arrowhead*) consistent with a type IV A choledochal cyst.

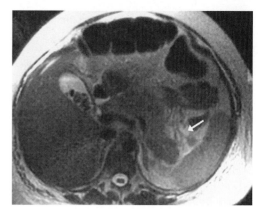

Fig. 9. Acute pancreatitis. Axial T2-weighted SSFSE image demonstrates an edematous pancreas with surrounding inflammation most prominent around the tail (*arrow*).

common on the right side and more pronounced during the late second and early third trimesters of pregnancy. The physiologic dilatation of the collecting system is asymptomatic most of the time; however, occasionally, patients can develop abdominal pain. In these cases, pathologic dilatation secondary to a stone or stricture must be excluded.

Urinary calculi affect 1 in 1500 pregnancies but account for most nonobstetric hospitalizations during gestation [1]. Most patients also present in late pregnancy, and differentiation from painful hydronephrosis of pregnancy without urolithiasis can be challenging.

US is the standard initial diagnostic test of choice for evaluation of hydronephrosis; however, assessment and visualization of the ureters are not adequate, especially in pregnant patients. Unenhanced magnetic resonance urography is a valuable and well- tolerated investigation for evaluation of painful hydronephrosis during pregnancy [42,43]. Spencer and colleagues [42] described the MR imaging findings of physiologic hydronephrosis as extrinsic compression of the middle third of the ureter, with a collapsed distal ureter and without any filling defect (Fig. 10). Conversely, perirenal fluid, a dilated ureter in the pelvis, and a filling defect inside the dilated ureter at the level of obstruction are reported as signs of pathologic hydronephrosis during pregnancy (most likely secondary to a stone) in magnetic resonance urography (Fig. 11) [42,43]. Thin-slice, high-resolution, highly T2-weighted FSE sequences improve the ability of magnetic resonance urography for detection of small stones. Care should be taken not to mistake air, clot, or flow artifacts for a stone.

Acute pyelonephritis occurs in 1% to 2% of pregnancies and usually results from asymptomatic bacteriuria or recurrent lower urinary tract infection

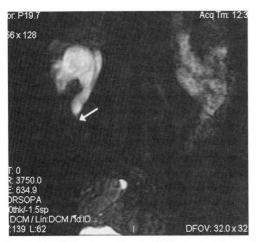

Fig. 10. Painful hydronephrosis of pregnancy. Coronal thin-slice, heavily T2-weighted, 3D FSE image shows significant hydronephrosis and hydroureter of the right kidney. The right ureter is dilated up to its mid-portion (*arrow*), where it is compressed by the gravid uterus. Incidentally noted is the double collecting system of the right kidney.

[44]. Symptoms during pregnancy are similar to those in the general population and include fever, flank pain, and nausea. Pyelonephritis is associated with premature labor [44]. Diagnosis is based on urinanalysis and urine cultures, and the initial therapy is usually empiric. Imaging is indicated in patients who do not respond to therapy or have recurrent pyelonephritis. MR imaging without intravenous contrast is not specific for diagnosis of acute pyelonephritis. An enlarged kidney with renal edema and associated perirenal fluid can be suggestive of acute pyelonephritis on noncontrast MR

images (Fig. 12) [11]. Complications of acute pyelonephritis, such as renal abscesses, can also be identified on MR images [45].

Gynecologic indications

Adnexal torsion

Adnexal torsion accounts for approximately 3% of gynecologic emergencies, and 20% to 25% of adnexal torsions occur in pregnant women [46]. It is one of the few causes of acute abdomen that is more common in pregnancy [2]. Torsion usually occurs between 6 and 14 weeks of gestation and commonly accompanies an ipsilateral ovarian neoplasm or cyst. Normal ovaries can also undergo torsion. In adnexal torsion, the ovary or the ipsilateral fallopian tube twists with the vascular pedicle, resulting in vascular compromise [47]. The presenting signs and symptoms are nonspecific and may include lateralized lower quadrant pain, nausea, vomiting, fever, lower quadrant tenderness, and a palpable adnexal mass. The diagnosis can be challenging. In pregnant patients, early diagnosis before tissue necrosis may allow ovary-sparing laparoscopic detorsion, followed by progesterone therapy if the corpus luteum is removed.

Gray-scale and color Doppler US have been reported to be useful in detecting adnexal torsion [47]. In challenging cases in which a definite diagnosis cannot be made by US, MR imaging can provide additional information to confirm the diagnosis [48]. On MR imaging, the ovary is enlarged with various sized follicles or a large mass. Findings of ovarian torsion on unenhanced MR images include a thick edematous pedicle, signal intensities indicative of hemorrhage within the ovary or

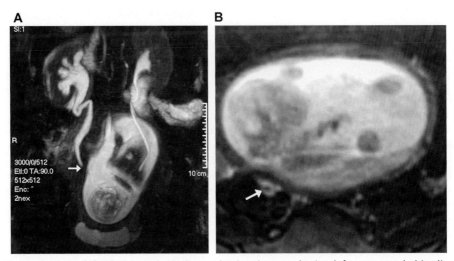

Fig. 11. Ureteral stone. (*A*) Maximum intensity projection image obtained from coronal thin-slice, heavily T2-weighted, 3D FSE images shows right hydronephrosis and hydroureter. (*B*) Level of the obstruction is distal (*arrow*), where a small stone is detected as a filling defect (*arrow*) on the axial T2-weighted FSE image.

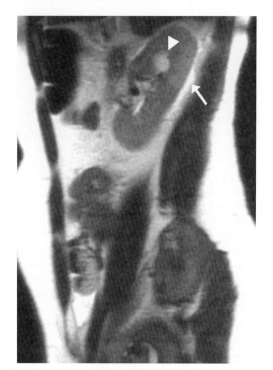

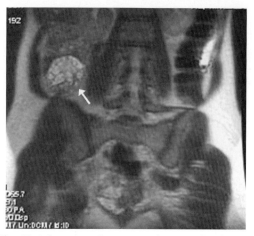

Fig. 13. Adnexal torsion. Coronal T2-weighted SSFSE image reveals an enlarged right ovary (*arrow*) containing multiple peripherally located follicles. This pregnant patient at 18 weeks of gestation had acute-onset right lower quadrant pain, and surgery confirmed the ovarian torsion.

Fig. 12. Acute pyelonephritis. Sagittal T2-weighted SSFSE image demonstrates focal hydronephrosis in the upper pole of the right kidney (*arrowhead*) and small amount of perinephric fluid around the upper pole (*arrow*). No stone or hydroureter is seen. The results of the urinanalysis were also compatible with pyelonephritis, and the patient was treated with antibiotics.

fallopian tube, and smooth wall thickening of the twisted ovarian cystic mass (Fig. 13) [47,49]. T1-weighted images are helpful to identify hemorrhage within the ovary as high signal intensity streaks [49]. Ascites and uterine deviation to the twisted side are other ancillary findings of ovarian torsion [47]. Lack of enhancement of the ovary after intravenous contrast administration may also allow diagnosis of ovarian torsion.

Leiomyomas

Uterine leiomyomas are found in approximately 2% of pregnant women, and 1 of 10 women have related complications during pregnancy [50]. Abdominal pain related to fibroids may be attributable to degeneration, rapid growth, or torsion. The major complication is hemorrhagic infarction (red degeneration), characterized by second- and early third-trimester pain, low-grade fever, and occasional bleeding [50]. Infarction usually involves the entire lesion and is secondary to obstruction of draining veins at the periphery of the lesion. Treatment consists of bedrest and nonsteroidal anti-inflammatory drugs [1].

MR imaging has been shown to be useful in characterizing uterine leiomyomas during pregnancy and contributes to an accurate diagnosis [51]. Degenerating leiomyomas typically exhibit high signal intensity on T2-weighted images and diffuse or peripheral high signal on T1-weighted images (Fig. 14) [8,52,53]. The peripheral rim, which has low signal intensity on T2-weighted images and high signal intensity on T1-weighted images, may correspond to the obstructed veins at the periphery of the mass [53]. On postcontrast images, there is lack of enhancement of the entire lesion.

Hemorrhagic cyst

Corpus luteum cysts may be recognized easily by US when they are not complicated [34]. Patients with bleeding into the cyst may present with abdominal pain and peritoneal signs. Their diagnosis by US is often challenging as a result of variations in size, thickness of the cyst wall, and internal echo pattern, depending on the formation and lysis of the clot [54]. On US, hemorrhagic cysts have been referred to as "the great imitator," and the differential diagnosis includes ectopic pregnancy, adnexal torsion, neoplasm, and pelvic inflammatory disease [54]. Treatment of hemorrhagic cysts is usually conservative, and such cysts must be differentiated from other conditions that may require immediate surgical intervention.

On MR imaging, corpus luteum cysts have thicker walls than follicular cysts. MR imaging can successfully detect the presence of hemorrhage into the cyst as intermediate to bright signal on T1- and

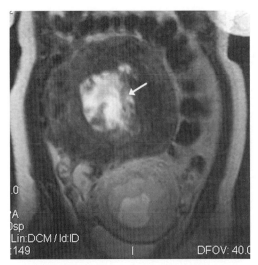

Fig. 14. Red degeneration of leiomyoma. Coronal T2-weighted SSFSE image shows a large exophytic fibroid superior to the gravid uterus with a central area of high intensity on the T2-weighted image (*arrow*), representing hemorrhagic necrosis. The patient's pain subsided with expectant therapy.

T2-weighted images that is not suppressed on fat-saturated sequences (Fig. 15). Acute hemorrhage may also have distinctly low intensity on T2-weighted images [55]. Hemoperitoneum can be recognized as high-intensity fluid on T1-weighted images. MR imaging may help to make a more specific diagnosis and save the patient from unnecessary surgery.

Adnexal masses
During the first trimester, the most common adnexal mass is the corpus luteum cyst, which usually regresses between weeks 10 and 15 of gestation [56]. Beyond the first trimester, most cystic masses are benign cystic teratomas or cystadenomas [34].

Adnexal masses can cause abdominal pain by compressing surrounding organs, torsion, tumoral bleeding, or rupture leading to peritonitis. Adnexal torsion should always be considered in a patient presenting with an adnexal mass and acute lower abdominal pain. Rupture of functional cysts, endometriomas, and benign and malignant neoplasms during pregnancy is rare but has been reported in the literature [57].

US remains the primary imaging tool in pregnant women who present with pelvic masses. If the results of US are equivocal, MR imaging can provide supplemental information that may influence patient treatment [56,58]. MR imaging can help in differentiating a fibroid from an ovarian neoplasm and can detect blood or fat within the tumor, enabling a more specific diagnosis (Fig. 16) [59].

Abdominal wall
Rectus sheath hematoma is a rare clinical entity that may present as acute abdominal pain. It is usually associated with abdominal trauma or anticoagulation therapy. It is often self-limiting but may lead to unnecessary laparotomy if the diagnosis is not recognized. Several case reports describing rectus sheath hematomas in pregnant patients have been reported, and some of the patients described required surgical exploration because of an inability to make a confident preoperative diagnosis [60]. US is a good screening technique but may be misleading at times, with a sensitivity as low as 50% [61]. MR imaging is useful in diagnosis of rectus sheath hematoma, which demonstrates a high signal intensity area on T1- and T2-weighted images (Fig. 17) [62]. Other pathologic conditions involving the abdominal wall, such as abscesses or hernias, are also successfully detected and characterized by MR imaging.

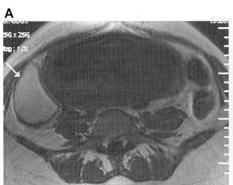
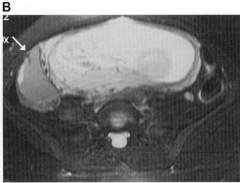

Fig. 15. Hemorrhagic cyst. (*A*) Axial T1-weighted FSE image shows a right ovarian cystic lesion (*arrow*) with bright signal. (*B*) The signal of the lesion (*arrow*) is not suppressed on the fat-saturated T2-weighted FSE image, consistent with a hemorrhagic cyst.

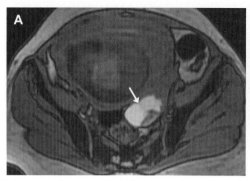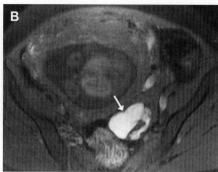

Fig. 16. Endometriosis. An ill-defined, predominantly bright-signal, heterogenous left adnexal mass (*arrow*) is seen on T1-weighted FSE (*A*) and fat-saturated T1-weighted FSE (*B*) images consistent with a hemorrhagic content. Acute abdominal pain of the patient subsided with expectant management. The patient underwent surgery after delivery, and histopathologic evaluation revealed endometriosis.

Obstetric indications

Ectopic pregnancy is a well-known potentially fatal acute condition associated with pregnancy. Ninety-five percent of ectopic pregnancies implant in the tubes, and the remainder implant in the uterine interstitium, cervix, ovaries, or elsewhere in the abdomen [63]. Transvaginal US in combination with quantitative serum assays of β-human chorionic gonadotropin (hCG) allow the diagnosis to be made. In some cases, a single US examination is not enough and serial follow-up of the patient with transvaginal US and serum β-hCG measurements is recommended. Surgery is the standard treatment of choice, but expectant management and medical treatment (systemic or local methotrexate injections) have emerged as therapeutic options during the past decade. A nonsurgical approach requires a highly accurate noninvasive test for the evaluation of patients with suspected ectopic pregnancy [64].

The role of MR imaging in diagnosis of ectopic pregnancy has not been clearly defined. It may be useful for diagnosis of rare or complicated forms, such as abdominal, interstitial, myometrial, or cervical pregnancy [65]. MR imaging findings of ectopic pregnancy include adnexal hematoma, gestational sac, heterogenous adnexal mass, dilated tubes, hemoperitoneum, and wall enhancement (Fig. 18) [65]. Kataoka and colleagues [64] reported that MR imaging allowed early diagnosis of ectopic pregnancy and enabled determination of the usefulness of early conservative therapy with methotrexate.

Subchorionic hemorrhage can cause bleeding and pain during pregnancy. It usually results in separation of the placenta from the myometrium and ranges from marginal subchorionic hemorrhage to placental abruption, in which the placenta separates from the myometrium prematurely. MR imaging can detect a small amount of blood posterior to the placenta as areas of high signal intensity on T1-weighted images [9,66]. MR imaging may differentiate hematomas of various ages from placental tissue [66].

Summary

MR imaging enables diagnosis of a variety of maternal diseases presenting as acute abdominal pain in

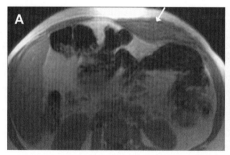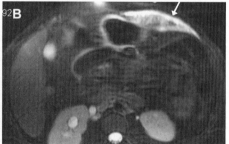

Fig. 17. Rectus sheath hematoma. (*A*) Axial T1-weighted GRE image demonstrates a thickened left rectus muscle (*arrow*) containing linear increased signal intensity. (*B*) Fat-saturated T2-weighted FSE sequence also shows bright signal in the thick left rectus muscle (*arrow*) consistent with rectus sheath hematoma.

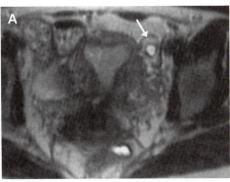 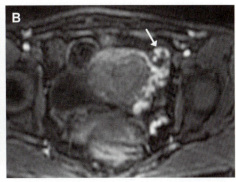

Fig. 18. Ectopic pregnancy. (*A*) Axial T2-weighted SSFSE image shows a well-defined cystic structure (*arrow*) in the left adnexa representing an extrauterine gestational sac. The left ovary can be seen separate from the sac on other images. (*B*) Postcontrast T1-weighted GRE image reveals avid enhancement of the wall of the gestational sac (*arrow*) as well as increased vascularity in the left adnexa. The patient was treated surgically, and the ectopic pregnancy was removed together with the left ovary and fallopian tube.

pregnant patients. When US is equivocal or non-diagnostic, MR imaging is a valuable complement to determine the exact etiology of acute abdominal pain. MR imaging often provides important information that influences patient management, and it is important for the radiologist to recognize the MR imaging appearance of common causes of acute abdominal pain during pregnancy.

References

[1] Cappell MS, Friedel D. Abdominal pain during pregnancy. Gastroenterol Clin North Am 2003; 32:1–58.

[2] Sharp HT. The acute abdomen during pregnancy. Clin Obstet Gynecol 2002;45:405–13.

[3] Oto A, Srinivasan PN, Ernst RD, et al. Revisiting MRI for appendix location during pregnancy. AJR Am J Roentgenol 2006;186:883–7.

[4] Lim HK, Bae SH, Seo GS. Diagnosis of acute appendicitis in pregnant women: value of sonography. AJR Am J Roentgenol 1992;159:539–42.

[5] Barloon TJ, Brown BP, Abu-Yousef MM, et al. Sonography of acute appendicitis in pregnancy. Abdom Imaging 1995;20:149–51.

[6] International Commission on Radiological Protection. Pregnancy and irradiation. Annals of the ICRP. Stockholm (Sweden): Elsevier Scientific; 2000. vol. 30: p. 1–43. Publication 84.

[7] Oto A, Srinivasan PN, Ernst RD, et al. Magnetic resonance imaging of maternal diseases causing acute abdominal pain during pregnancy: a pictorial review. J Comput Assist Tomogr 2005;29: 408–14.

[8] Brown MA, Birchard KB, Semelka RC. MR evaluation of pregnant patients with acute abdominal pain. Semin Ultrasound CT MR 2005;26:206–11.

[9] Eyvazzadeh AD, Pedrosa I, Rofsky NM, et al. MRI of right-sided abdominal pain in pregnancy. AJR Am J Roentgenol 2004;183(4):907–14.

[10] Cobben LP, Groot I, Haans L, et al. MRI for clinically suspected appendicitis during pregnancy. AJR Am J Roentgenol 2004;183:671–5.

[11] Birchard KR, Brown MA, Hyslop WB, et al. MRI of acute abdominal and pelvic pain in pregnant patients. AJR Am J Roentgenol 2005;184:452–8.

[12] Oto A, Ernst RD, Shah R, et al. Right-lower-quadrant pain and suspected appendicitis in pregnant women: evaluation with MR imaging—initial experience. Radiology 2005;234:445–51.

[13] Pedrosa I, Levine D, Eyvazzadeh AD, et al. MR imaging evaluation of acute appendicitis in pregnancy. Radiology 2006;238(3):891–9.

[14] Shellock FG, Kanal E. Policies, guidelines, and recommendations for MR imaging safety and patient management. SMRI Safety Committee. J Magn Reson Imaging 1991;1:97–101.

[15] De Wilde JP, Rivers AW, Price DL. A review of the current use of magnetic resonance imaging in pregnancy and safety implications for the fetus. Prog Biophys Mol Biol 2005;87(2–3):335–53.

[16] Kok RD, de Vries MM, Heerschap A, et al. Absence of harmful effects of magnetic resonance exposure at 1.5T in utero during the third trimester of pregnancy: a follow-up study. Magn Reson Imaging 2004;22(6):851–4.

[17] Baker PN, Johnson IR, Harvey PR, et al. A three-year follow-up of children imaged in utero with echo-planar magnetic resonance. Am J Obstet Gynecol 1994;170:32–3.

[18] Myers C, Duncan KR, Gowland PA, et al. Failure to detect intrauterine growth restriction following in utero exposure to MRI. Br J Radiol 1998; 71(845):549–51.

[19] Clements H, Duncan KR, Fielding K, et al. Infants exposed to MRI in utero have a normal paediatric assessment at 9 months of age. Br J Radiol 2000;73(866):190–4.

[20] US Food and Drug Administration. Magnetic resonance diagnostic device: panel recommendation and report on petitions for MR classification. Federal Register 1988;53:7575–9.

[21] Baer JL, Reis RA, Arens RA. Appendicitis in pregnancy with changes in position and axis of normal appendix in pregnancy. JAMA 1932;98:1359–64.

[22] Incesu L, Coskun A, Selcuk MB, et al. Acute appendicitis: MR imaging and sonographic correlation. AJR Am J Roentgenol 1997;168:669–74.

[23] Hormann M, Paya K, Eibenberger K, et al. MR imaging in children with nonperforated acute appendicitis: value of unenhanced MR imaging in sonographically selected cases. AJR Am J Roentgenol 1998;171:467–70.

[24] Firstenberg MS, Malangoni MA. Gastrointestinal surgery during pregnancy. Gastroenterol Clin North Am 1998;27:73–88.

[25] Wanetick LH, Roschen FP, Dunn JM. Volvulus of the small bowel complicating pregnancy. J Reprod Med 1975;14(2):82–3.

[26] Regan F, Beall DP, Bohlman ME, et al. Fast MR Imaging and the detection of small bowel obstruction. AJR Am J Roentgenol 1998;170(6):1465–9.

[27] Mogadam M, Korelitz BI, Ahmed SW, et al. The course of inflammatory bowel disease during pregnancy and postpartum. Am J Gastroenterol 1981;5(4):265–9.

[28] Hanan IM. Inflammatory bowel disease in the pregnant woman. Compr Ther 1993;19:91–5.

[29] Ferrero S, Ragni N. Inflammatory bowel disease: management issues during pregnancy. Arch Gynecol Obstet 2004;27:79–85.

[30] Horthuis K, Lavini Mphil C, Stoker J. MRI in Crohn's disease. J Magn Reson Imaging 2005;22(1):1–12.

[31] Shoenut JP, Semelka RC, Silverman R, et al. MRI in the diagnosis of Crohn's disease in two pregnant women. J Clin Gastroenterol 1993;17:244–7.

[32] Maccioni F, Viscido A, Broglia L, et al. Evaluation of Crohn disease activity with magnetic resonance imaging. Abdom Imaging 2000;25(3):219–28.

[33] Van bodegraven AA, Bohmer CJ, Manoliu RA, et al. Gallbladder contents and fasting gallbladder volumes during and after pregnancy. Scand J Gastroenterol 1998;33(9):993–7.

[34] El-Shawarby SA, Hendeson AF, Mossa MA. Ovarian cysts during pregnancy: dilemmas in diagnosis and management. J Obstet Gynaecol 2005;25(7):669–75.

[35] Adusumilli S, Siegelman ES. MR imaging of the gallbladder. Magn Reson Imaging Clin N Am 2002;10:165–84.

[36] Regan F, Schaefer DC, Smith DP, et al. The diagnostic utility of HASTE MRI in the evaluation of acute cholecystitis. Half-Fourier acquisition single-shot turbo SE. J Comput Assist Tomogr 1998;22(4):638–42.

[37] Griffin N, Wastle ML, Dunn WK, et al. Magnetic resonance cholangiopancreatography versus endoscopic retrograde cholangiopancreatography in the diagnosis of choledocholithiasis. Eur J Gastroenterol Hepatol 2003;15(7):809–13.

[38] Masui T, Katayama M, Kobayashi S, et al. Magnetic resonance cholangiopancreatography: comparison of respiratory-triggered three-dimensional fast-recovery fast spin-echo with parallel imaging technique and breath-hold half-Fourier two-dimensional single-shot fast spin-echo technique. Radiat Med 2006;24(3):202–9.

[39] Shanley DJ, Gagliardi JA, Daum-Kowalski R. Choledochal cyst complicating pregnancy: antepartum diagnosis with MRI. Abdom Imaging 1994;19(1):61–3.

[40] Ramin KD, Ramin SM, Richey SD, et al. Acute pancreatitis in pregnancy. Am J Obstet Gynecol 1995;173(1):187–91.

[41] Miller FH, Keppke AL, Dalal K, et al. MRI of pancreatitis and its complications: part 1, acute pancreatitis. AJR Am J Roentgenol 2004;183(6):1637–44.

[42] Spencer JA, Chahal R, Kelly A, et al. Evaluation of painful hydronephrosis in pregnancy: magnetic resonance urographic patterns in physiological dilatation versus calculous obstruction. J Urol 2004;171:256–60.

[43] Roy C, Saussine C, LeBras Y, et al. Assessment of painful ureterohydronephrosis during pregnancy by MR urography. Eur Radiol 1996;6(3):334–8.

[44] Millar LK, Cox SM. Urinary tract infections complicating pregnancy. Infect Dis Clin North Am 1997;11(1):13–26.

[45] Brown ED, Brown JJ, Kettritz U, et al. Renal abscesses: appearance on gadolinium-enhanced magnetic resonance images. Abdom Imaging 1996;21(2):172–6.

[46] McGowan L. Surgical diseases of the ovary in pregnancy. Clin Obstet Gynecol 1983;26(4):843–52.

[47] Rha SE, Byun JY, Jung SE, et al. CT and MR imaging features of adnexal torsion. Radiographics 2002;22:283–94.

[48] Nishino M, Hayakawa K, Iwasaku K, et al. Magnetic resonance imaging findings in gynecologic emergencies. J Comput Assist Tomogr 2003;27:564–70.

[49] Born C, Wirth S, Stabler A, et al. Diagnosis of adnexal torsion in the third trimester of pregnancy: a case report. Abdom Imaging 2004;29:123–7.

[50] Katz VL, Dotters DJ, Droegemeuller W. Complications of uterine leiomyomas in pregnancy. Obstet Gynecol 1989;73(4):593–6.

[51] Sherer DM, Maitland CY, Levine NF, et al. Prenatal magnetic resonance imaging assisting in differentiating between large degenerating intramural leiomyoma and a complex adnexal mass during pregnancy. Matern Fetal Med 2000;9(3):186–9.

[52] Ueda H, Togashi K, Konishi I, et al. Unusual appearances of uterine leiomyomas: MR imaging findings and their histopathologic backgrounds. Radiographics 1999;19:S131–45.

[53] Kawakami S, Togashi K, Konishi I, et al. Red degeneration of uterine leiomyoma: MR

appearance. J Comput Assist Tomogr 1994; 18(6):925–8.

[54] Swire MN, Castro-Aragon I, Levine D. Various sonographic appearances of the hemorrhagic corpus luteum cyst. Ultrasound Q 2004;20:45–58.

[55] Tamai K, Koyama T, Saga T. et al. MR features of physiologic and benign conditions of the ovary. Eur Radiol 2006;16:2700–11; [Epub ahead of print].

[56] Kier R, McCarthy SM, Scoutt LM, et al. Pelvic masses in pregnancy: MR imaging. Radiology 1990;176:709–13.

[57] Garcia-Velasco JA, Alvarez M, Palumbo A, et al. Rupture of an ovarian endometrioma during the first trimester of pregnancy. Eur J Obstet Gynecol Reprod Biol 1998;76(1):41–3.

[58] Weinreb JC, Brown CE, Lowe TW, et al. Pelvic masses in pregnant patients: MR and US imaging. Radiology 1986;159(3):717–24.

[59] Imaoka I, Wada A, Kaji Y, et al. Developing an MR imaging strategy for diagnosis of ovarian masses. Radiographics 2006;26(5):1431–48.

[60] Ramirez MM, Burkhead JM 3rd, Turrentine MA. Spontaneous rectus sheath hematoma during pregnancy mimicking abruption placenta. Am J Perinatol 1997;14(6):321–3.

[61] Khan MI, Medhat O, Popescu O, et al. Rectus sheath hematoma presenting as acute abdomen. ANZ J Surg 2005;75(6):502–3.

[62] Fukuda T, Sakamoto I, Kohzaki S, et al. Spontaneous rectus sheath hematomas: clinical and radiological features. Abdom Imaging 1996;21(1): 58–61.

[63] Salzberg MR. Ectopic pregnancy. N Engl J Med 1994;330(10):713–4.

[64] Kataoka ML, Togashi K, Kobayashi H, et al. Evaluation of ectopic pregnancy by magnetic resonance imaging. Hum Reprod 1999;14(10):2644–50.

[65] Nagayama M, Watanabe Y, Okumura A, et al. Fast MR imaging in obstetrics. Radiographics 2002;22(3):563–80.

[66] Trop I, Levine D. Hemorrhage during pregnancy: sonography and MR imaging. AJR Am J Roentgenol 2001;176(3):607–615.

ELSEVIER
SAUNDERS

MAGNETIC
RESONANCE
IMAGING CLINICS

Magn Reson Imaging Clin N Am 14 (2007) 503–522

Fetal MR Imaging

Rosalind B. Dietrich, MD*, Inbal Cohen, MD

- Safety
- Technique
- Normal fetal brain development
- Indications for fetal MR imaging
  Evaluation of abnormalities of ventricular size and shape
  Agenesis of the corpus callosum
  Other developmental anomalies

Posterior fossa anomalies: is there a Dandy-Walker malformation?
Fluid collections and mass lesions
Is there a destructive brain lesion or the presence of hemorrhage?
Is spinal dysraphism present?
Increased risk of anomalies being present
- Summary
- References

Ultrasonography is the primary prenatal screening modality used in the evaluation of the fetus and the maternal pelvis. In most cases studied, ultrasonography produces excellent images, and detects any fetal anomalies present and clearly defines them. Occasionally, however, complete evaluation of the fetus is not possible because of technical problems. These problems may occur when oligohydramnios or maternal obesity is present, or if the fetus is in a position that makes it difficult to image technically. In some instances, acoustic shadowing from the ossified calvaria may obscure detail of part of the fetal brain. In other instances, ultrasound may detect an abnormality but more information is needed in order to reach a definitive diagnosis so that appropriate counseling can be given.

The inherently higher contrast resolution of fetal MR imaging, its large field of view, and its ability to visualize directly both sides of the fetal brain enable it to better define fetal brain anatomy and pathology. Although early images were limited because of fetal motion, the development of new, faster, single-slice imaging sequences and parallel imaging have enabled radiologists to obtain single-slice images in less than 1 second, making it possible to obtain images of a moving fetus. As a result of these developments, fetal MR imaging is now being used increasingly as a complementary technique in the evaluation the fetal brain [1–6].

Several studies have been reported comparing sonography and fetal MR imaging in groups of fetuses with suspected anomalies of the brain and spine. These studies found that in a significant number of cases, MR imaging defined anatomic detail better, changed the diagnosis, and subsequently guided management decisions [7–13]. In addition, fetal MR imaging may help identify those patients who would benefit from prenatal intervention, and aid in their fetal surgical planning [14].

Safety

Interpretation of the studies performed to evaluate the safety of MR imaging during pregnancy is problematic. Although data on MR safety in pregnant animals and animal embryos are available, few studies evaluating the safety of MR in humans have been performed [15]. These studies include several that demonstrated no long-term adverse

Department of Radiology, University of California, San Diego Medical Center, 200 West Arbor Drive, San Diego, CA 92103, USA
* Corresponding author.
E-mail address: rdietrich@ucsd.edu (R.B. Dietrich).

effects from fetal MR in children who were imaged as fetuses [16–19], one study showing no increase in adverse pregnancy outcomes in female MR imaging workers [20], and one study showing no increased incidence of growth restriction in the fetuses of mothers undergoing MR imaging during pregnancy [21]. Unfortunately, the information from these studies is limited because often they were performed using different field strength magnets and gradients on patients at differing gestational ages. Fetal MR imaging is not a screening tool and, although the literature implies no apparent danger, it should be used only in cases of recognized or strongly suspected abnormalities. In such cases, it is generally believed that the small potential risk is outweighed by the benefit of the additional information that can be obtained [22].

Despite this, fetal MR imaging is performed rarely before 18 to 20 weeks of gestation, and is never performed during the period of organogenesis, when the theoretic risk would be greatest. Informed consent should always be obtained before the start of the study.

Technique

Patients undergoing fetal MR imaging are asked to remain NPO for several hours before the study, to decrease fetal motion. At the authors' institution, studies are obtained on a 1.5 Tesla magnet using a (four-element) phased-array pelvic coil. The patient is positioned in the magnet in a supine or a left posterior oblique position, and 3-D, large, field-of-view scout images are obtained of the mother's pelvis, to localize the orientation of the fetus and ensure that the coil is positioned to give maximum possible signal intensity to the area of study. Despite this, the fetus and the receiver coil

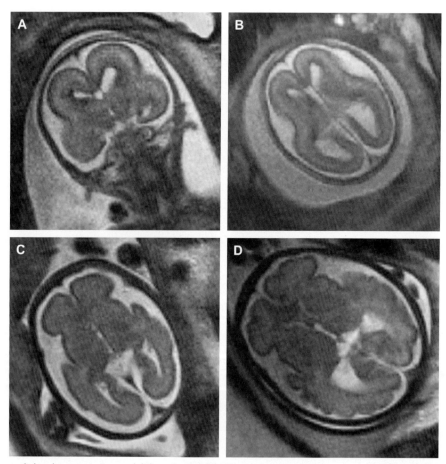

Fig. 1. Normal development. Coronal (*A*) and axial (*B*) T2-weighted HASTE images of a 22-week fetus demonstrate smooth appearance of the brain cortex, with shallow sylvian fissures and layers of varying signal intensity within the cerebral hemispheres. On axial T2-weighted HASTE image at 27 weeks (*C*), the sylvian fissures have a more squared appearance. Axial T2-weighted HASTE image at 30 weeks (*D*) shows further development of the sulcal-gyral pattern.

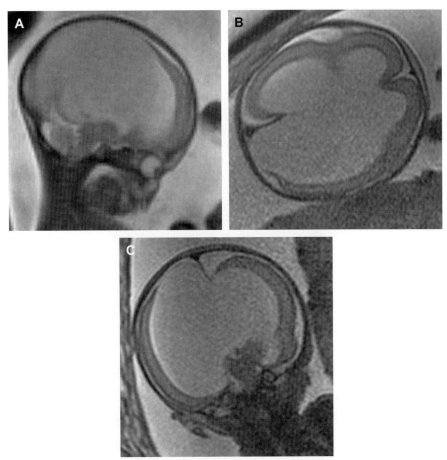

Fig. 2. Ventriculomegaly-aqueductal stenosis. Sagittal (*A*), axial (*B*), and coronal (*C*) T2-weighted HASTE images demonstrate markedly dilated lateral ventricles. The fourth ventricle is normal in size (*A*). The cortical mantle is thinned, and a portion of the left mantle (*B*, *C*) is absent posteriorly.

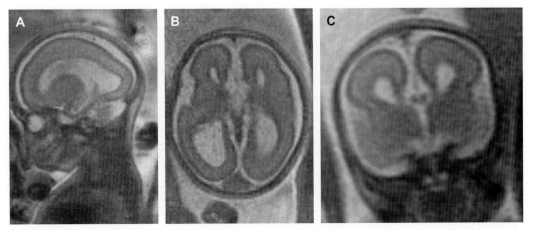

Fig. 3. Absence of the corpus callosum. Sagittal (*A*), axial (*B*), and coronal (*C*) T2-weighted HASTE images in a 31-week gestation show absence of the corpus callosum. On the axial image, the lateral ventricles have a parallel configuration and colpocephaly is present. Coronal image (*C*) shows the frontal horns have a "stag-horn" appearance and no white matter fibers cross the midline.

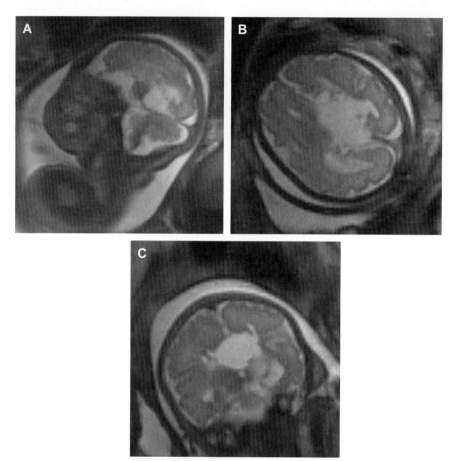

Fig. 4. Absence of the corpus callosum with interhemispheric cyst. Sagittal (*A*), axial (*B*), and coronal (*C*) T2-weighted HASTE images in a 31-week gestation show a lobulated, midline cyst extending superiorly from the region of the third ventricle. The corpus callosum is absent.

may still be far apart, making visualization of small structures difficult. Occasionally, the coil may need to be repositioned during the study to image the whole fetus optimally.

Images are obtained routinely of the fetal head and body in three orthogonal planes, using ultra-fast MR techniques. Each subsequent image sequence is prescribed in a plane orthogonal to the preceding set. Slice thicknesses range from 2 to 4 mm, with no gap between slices. The field of view selected should be as small as possible; it varies, depending on the size of the fetus and the fetal area being studied, but is usually between 220 and 320 mm. The smallness of the field of view that can be obtained may be limited by aliasing and wrap artifacts. In most cases, T2-weighted sequences are obtained during quiet respiration using the half-Fourier acquired single-shot turbo spin-echo (HASTE) (TR 1100, TE 114, 1 average), and the true fast imaging with steady-state free precession technique (FISP) (TR 4.4, TE 2.2, 1 average) sequences [23]. Subsequently, 2-D and 3-D FISP sequences are obtained

through the fetus. T1-weighted sequences are obtained using a fast, multiplanar, gradient-echo technique as well, when destructive or hemorrhagic lesions are suspected, or to visualize the position of the liver and meconium-filled bowel loops [24,25]. Because these take considerably longer to obtain, (20–45 seconds), breath-hold techniques may be used. Because most sequences take less than 25 seconds, the total examination time is around 30 minutes.

Additional techniques are beginning to be used in some centers; these include gradient-echo echo-planar T2*WI to evaluate for hemorrhage [26], diffusion imaging to evaluate water motion patterns in congenital anomalies and ischemic lesions [27,28], and cine MR imaging to evaluate fetal motion [29]. The potential role of MR spectroscopy in the evaluation of the fetal brain is being evaluated [30–35]. Because of the large voxel size and long acquisition times required, its current use in the fetus is limited to the third trimester, when movement is more limited because the fetal head is engaged.

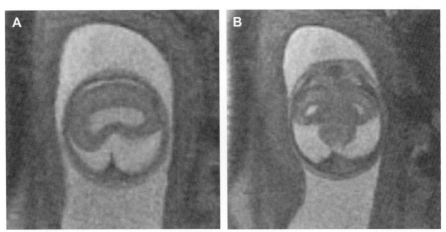

Fig. 5. Alobar holoprosencephaly. Axial T2-weighted HASTE images (*A*, *B*) show a saucer-like rim of cerebral tissue anteriorly containing a monoventricle (*A*). The hemispheres are not separated and the septum pellucidum is absent. A dorsal cyst is present and the thalami are fused completely (*B*).

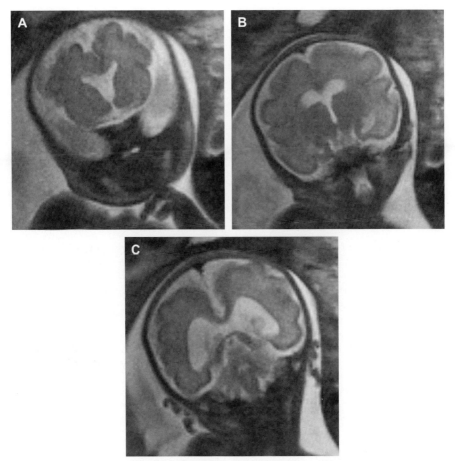

Fig. 6. Semilobar holoprosencephaly with midsegment interhemispheric fusion. Coronal T2-weighted HASTE images (*A*, *B*, *C*) demonstrate complete absence of the septum pellucidum. Partial agenesis of the midportion of the corpus callosum is seen, with fusion of cerebral hemispheres across the midline in this region (*B*).

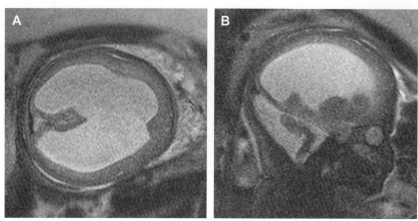

Fig. 7. Walker-Warburg syndrome with marked dilatation of lateral ventricles. Axial (*A*) and sagittal (*B*) T2-weighted HASTE images show that the cortex is smooth and the sylvian fissures are not developed (*A*). The posterior fossa is small and the cerebellar hemispheres are severely hypoplastic (*B*).

Normal fetal brain development

One of the advantages of fetal MR imaging over prenatal ultrasonography is its ability to visualize the surface anatomy of the brain. Several articles in the literature describe in detail the changing MR appearance of both the supratentorial fetal brain and the posterior fossa structures during their development [26,36–44]. Using established criteria, the maturity of the fetal brain can be assessed accurately by evaluating the sulcal pattern and the appearance of the migrating cell layers. Before 18 weeks of gestation, the surface of the fetal brain is smooth, and the sylvian fissure appears as a smooth, shallow indentation on its surface (Fig. 1); by 23 weeks, the sylvian fissure demonstrates a more squared

appearance. As the fetus matures, other primary sulci appear in an orderly progression on the surface of the brain, and gradually become deeper. Later, these are followed by the development of secondary and tertiary sulci. The timing of the appearance of each sulcus is very specific and enables precise information to be obtained on the maturity of the fetus. Normally, a slight asymmetry in the appearance of the sulci may be seen and a delay of sulcal formation may present in twin pregnancies. The timing of the initial identification of the various sulci on MR images lags 1 to 2 weeks behind when they can first be seen on fetal autopsy specimens [38,40].

During the second and early third trimesters, several layers of differing signal intensities can be

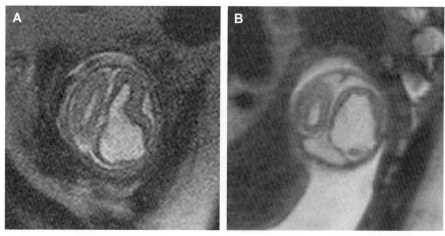

Fig. 8. Hemimegalencephaly. Axial (*A*) and coronal (*B*) T2-weighted HASTE images show an enlarged left hemisphere containing a large lateral ventricle.

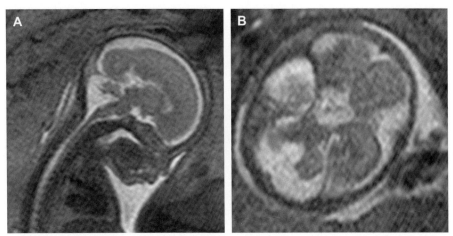

Fig. 9. Dandy-Walker variant (inferior cerebellar hypoplasia). Sagittal (*A*) and axial (*B*) T2-weighted HASTE images at 21 weeks of gestation demonstrate an enlarged posterior fossa. The inferior portion of the vermis is absent and the cerebellar hemispheres are hypoplastic. A retrocerebellar cyst communicates with the fourth ventricle.

seen on T2-weighted HASTE sequences (see Fig. 1). The future gray matter or cortical plate has the appearance of a low signal intensity ribbon along the periphery of the brain. A dark band of low T2 signal intensity is also seen bordering the lateral ventricles, and represents the germinal matrix (or ventricular zone). Early in gestation, the germinal matrix completely surrounds the lateral ventricles, but regresses during the third trimester, until at term it is seen only in the region of the caudo-thalamic groove. The remainder of the brain parenchyma between these two T2-dark bands has higher signal intensity. Several different layers may be identified within it, which represent the peri-ventricular, subventricular, and intermediate zones, and the subplate [26]. These layers can also be identified on T1-weighted images [36,41].

The corpus callosum develops between the eighth and twentieth weeks of gestation and is seen on T2-weighted images as a low intensity structure with uniform thickness throughout the fetal life. It is seen most easily on coronal images as a low intensity band, crossing the midline above the lateral ventricles and cavum septi pellucidi.

The anatomy of brain stem and cerebellum are also well seen on fetal MR. Compared with the term infant, in the fetus the cerebellum is relatively smaller than the cerebrum, and the pericerebellar fluid spaces are more prominent. On sagittal images, the pontine curvature and bulbar sulcus can be seen, and the triangular-shaped fourth ventricle is covered completely by the cerebellar vermis [44]. Because the cerebellar fissures are very thin compared with the slice thickness, the cerebellar fissures are seen poorly on fetal MR images. However,

the primary fissure (which separates the anterior lobe from the posterior lobe) usually can be seen by 25 to 26 weeks of gestation, and is always seen by 28 weeks [44]. By 33 to 37 weeks of gestation, the remainder of the hemispheric fissures are seen better. On fast T2-weighted sequences, the cerebellar cortex and the central dentate nuclei have low signal intensity, compared with the intervening white matter, which has relatively higher signal intensity because of its higher cellularity [44]. Because the cerebellum increases in size later in gestation, transverse cerebellar measurements and volumetric assessment can be used to help assess normal cerebellar development in the third trimester [45,46].

Fetal MR imaging can show the size and shape of the lateral ventricles clearly. Although good correlation between ultrasound and MR imaging ventricular measurements have been shown [47], ventricular measurements probably are assessed better using ultrasonography because normative values are more established using this technique. In the fetus, the ventricles have smooth walls throughout gestation and are considered normal in size when they measure less than 10 mm (measured along the posterior choroid plexus on axial images obtained at the level of the thalami). A recent study evaluating the size of the ventricles during fetal life showed that ventricular volume does not vary with gestational age, whereas cerebral and cerebellar volumes increase significantly [48]. Ventricles that measure more than 10 mm are therefore considered abnormal.

Before 32 to 34 weeks of gestation, the fetal sub-arachnoid spaces appear prominent on MR images.

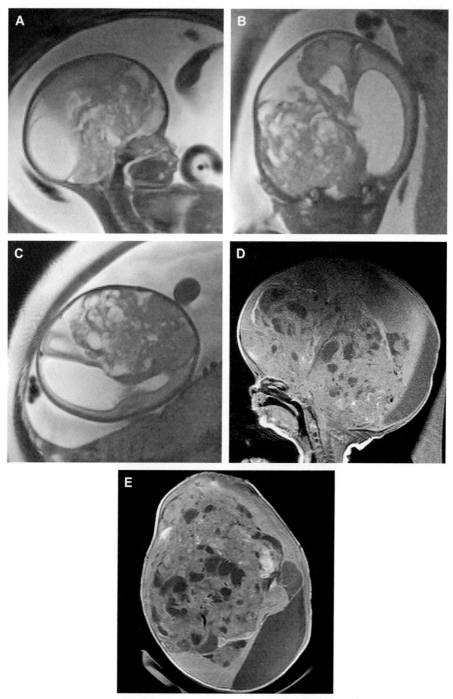

Fig. 10. Intracranial teratoma. Sagittal (*A*), coronal (*B*), and axial (*C*) T2-weighted HASTE images at 28 weeks of gestation show a heterogenous signal intensity mass filling the anterior and middle cranial fossae, compressing the ipsilateral hemisphere and obstructing the contralateral lateral ventricle. Sagittal (*D*) and Axial (*E*) T1-weighted images obtained after birth show that the lobulated, heterogenous mass has increased in size; compresses the right cerebrum, brain stem, and cerebellum; and causes obstructive hydrocephalus.

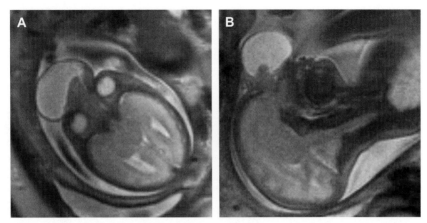

Fig. 11. Frontoethmoidal meningo-encephalocele. Axial (*A*) and sagittal (*B*) T2-weighted HASTE images at 22 weeks of gestation demonstrate a circumscribed, thin-walled mass extending though a defect in the frontoethmoidal bones. It contains CSF, leptomeninges, and neural tissue.

After this time, they begin to decrease in size, starting first in the subarachnoid space anterior to the frontal lobes (32 weeks), and slightly later adjacent to the parietal lobes (34 weeks) [49]. This decrease in size continues until term.

Indications for fetal MR imaging

In the following section the authors discuss some of the more frequent indications for fetal MR imaging.

Evaluation of abnormalities of ventricular size and shape

Evaluation of ventriculomegaly, which has been seen previously by prenatal ultrasonography, is the most common indication for fetal MR. Usually, the MR imaging study is performed to evaluate the size and the shape of the ventricles further, and to determine if other associated abnormalities are present. As on ultrasound studies, the lateral ventricles are measured routinely at the posterior margin of the choroid plexus on axial images obtained at the level of the thalami; ventricles that measure more than 10 mm are considered abnormal. Although abnormally large ventricles can be seen in various disorders, it is reported that 50% of cases of isolated hydrocephalus are caused by the presence of a Chiari II malformation, aqueductal stenosis (Fig. 2), or a Dandy-Walker malformation [4]. Other causes include developmental supratentorial anomalies, such as absence or hypoplasia of the corpus callosum, and migrational disorders, such as lissencephaly and holoprosencephalies. Asymmetrically enlarged ventricles can be seen in schizencephaly and hemimegalencephaly, and in destructive disorders.

Knowledge of the cause of the hydrocephalus and whether associated anomalies are present can

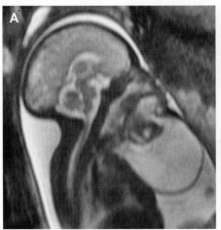
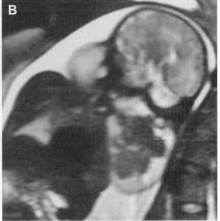

Fig. 12. Cystic hygroma. Sagittal (*A*) and oblique (*B*) T2-weighted HASTE images at 35 weeks of gestation show a multicystic neck mass extending into the chin and lower lip.

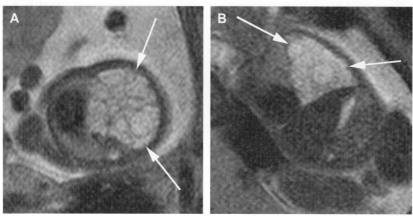

Fig. 13. CCAM type 2. Axial (*A*) and coronal (*B*) T2-weighted HASTE images at 21 weeks gestation show that a cystic mass completely fills the left hemithorax (*arrows*) and displaces the heart and mediastinum to the right.

be useful to clinicians and patients. Although it seems clear that most cases of severe hydrocephalus seen on fetal MR imaging have a guarded prognosis [50], it is far from clear what the prognosis is for fetuses with milder forms of isolated ventriculomegaly [51–54]. Poor neurologic outcome is associated more often with an atrial width greater than or equal to 12 mm, asymmetric bilateral enlargement, and progression of ventriculomegaly [52].

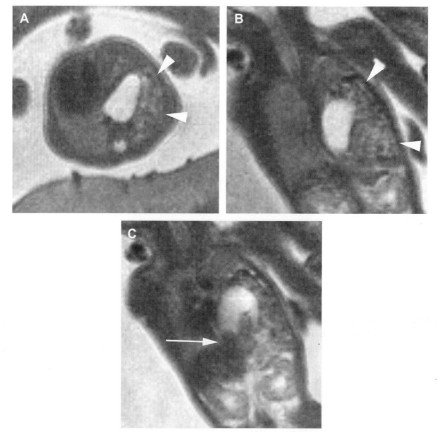

Fig. 14. Left congenital diaphragmatic hernia. Axial (*A*) and coronal (*B, C*) T2-weighted HASTE images at 22 weeks gestation show a large mass (*white arrowheads*) containing the stomach, bowel, and a portion of the left lobe of the liver (*white arrow*), which are herniating into the left hemithorax, causing mediastinal shift.

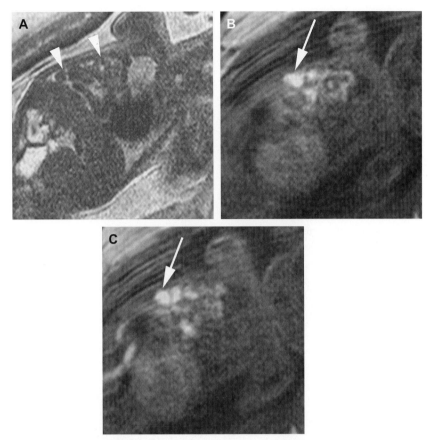

Fig. 15. Left congenital diaphragmatic hernia. Coronal (*A*) T2-weighted HASTE image shows multiple loops of bowel and part of the stomach (*arrowheads*) herniating into the left hemithorax, causing displacement of the mediastinum. Coronal T1-weighted images (*B*, *C*) confirm the diagnosis by showing bright, meconium-filled bowel loops in the chest (*arrows*).

Agenesis of the corpus callosum

MR imaging is useful in the evaluation of fetuses suspected of having callosal anomalies on prenatal ultrasound studies. Although the suspicion of callosal abnormality may be raised by ultrasound, often it is based on indirect signs, because it is difficult technically to directly image midline structures sagittally using this modality. MR imaging is superior in its ability to directly visualize the corpus callosum, which is visualized best on coronal images obtained after 20 weeks of gestation. MR can visualize a normal corpus callosum in 20% of patients with a suspicious ultrasound study, information that is very reassuring to parents [55]. Direct visualization enables differentiation of total agenesis, partial agenesis, and hypoplasia of the corpus callosum (Fig. 3). MR imaging can also identify the presence of associated interhemispheric cysts and lipomas (Fig. 4) [56,57]. Fetal MR can detect associated central nervous system abnormalities that may be occult sonographically in up to 63% of cases [55].

Such abnormalities include Dandy-Walker malformation, Chiari II malformation, gray matter heterotopia, holoprosencephaly, schizencephaly, and encephalocele [58]. Patients who have callosal anomalies may be asymptomatic or have clinical symptoms such as seizures, psychotic disorders, or intellectual impairment; those with associated anomalies are more likely to be symptomatic.

Other developmental anomalies

Other developmental anomalies, such as holoprosencephaly and migrational disorders, may be diagnosed by fetal MR imaging following a referral for evaluation of ventriculomegaly. In fetuses with holoprosencephaly, MR images show a small or normal-sized head and an absence of normal midline anatomy [59–61]. In addition, they may demonstrate a monoventricle or dorsal cyst (Figs. 5 and 6).

Fetal MR is useful particularly in the diagnosis of migrational disorders because prenatal ultrasonography is unable to demonstrate the anatomy of the cortical sulcal-gyral pattern [62–65]. After 25

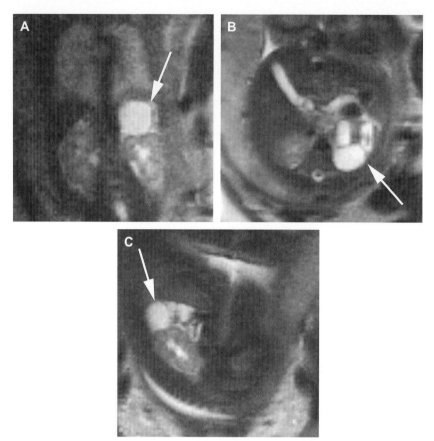

Fig. 16. Cystic neuroblastoma. Coronal (*A*), axial (*B*), and sagittal (*C*) T2-weighted HASTE images were obtained at 19 weeks of gestation and show a cystic adrenal mass (*arrows*).

weeks of gestation, MR is able to demonstrate the appearance of the normal cortical landmarks [62]. Absence of, or a delay in, the development of these landmarks raises the suspicion of the presence of a migrational disorder (Fig. 7). Thus, MR can be helpful in the diagnosis of lissencephaly, schizencephaly, polymicrogyria, heterotopic gray matter, and hemimegalencephaly (Fig. 8) [28,62].

Posterior fossa anomalies: is there a Dandy-Walker malformation?

Evaluation of the posterior fossa may be difficult using ultrasound. Fetal MR may be helpful in confirming the presence of cystic abnormalities, such as Dandy-Walker malformations, mega cisterna magna, and arachnoid cysts, and in differentiating them [66]. As fetal MR techniques improve, increasingly subtle vermian and hemispheric anomalies may be identified [67].

Often, fetal MR imaging is ordered when prenatal ultrasound raises the question of the presence of a Dandy-Walker malformation or variant being present. Sagittal and axial images can show the size and shape of the cerebellar vermis clearly, demonstrate the tecto-vermian angle, and evaluate the cerebellar hemispheres and brainstem (Fig. 9). Although the identification of a Dandy-Walker malformation is often helpful to perinatologists and parents as major decisions about continuation or termination of a pregnancy are made, the discovery of inferior vermian hypoplasia (or a Dandy-Walker variant) can cause problems for counselors because its clinical significance is not understood completely.

A recent paper reported the postnatal imaging findings and neurodevelopmental outcome in 19 subjects in whom a diagnosis of inferior vermian hypoplasia was made on fetal MR imaging examination [67]. The investigators found that, although the diagnosis was confirmed on postnatal imaging in 68% of cases, 32% had normal postnatal imaging. On developmental testing performed between 14 and 24 months of age, 23% had motor and language delays and 15% had behavioral problems.

More recently, several investigators have reported the use of fetal MR imaging in the detection

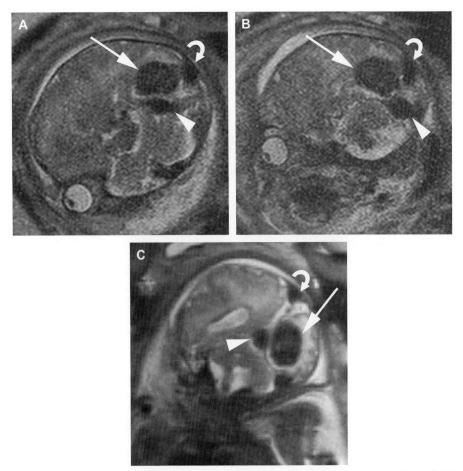

Fig. 17. Supratentorial hematoma. Fetal MR imaging study at 39 weeks of gestation was performed following an abnormal fetal ultrasound that showed severe oligohydramnios and ascites. Sagittal (*A, B*), true FISP, and coronal HASTE (*C*) images show a low signal intensity posterior right intracerebral hematoma (*arrow*) with surrounding edema. Additionally, the superior sagittal sinus (*curved arrow*) and straight sinus (*arrowhead*) are dilated with low signal intensity, possibly caused by dural sinus thrombosis in association with fetal hydrops.

of less common posterior fossa anomalies, such as rhombencephalosynapsis, in patients who have severe hypoplasia of the brainstem, and in patients who have vermian hypoplasia in association with Joubert's syndrome [68–71].

Fluid collections and mass lesions

The identification by prenatal ultrasonography of a large fluid collection or a mass lesion may be an indication for fetal MR imaging. MR imaging can differentiate intra-axial, extra-axial, and extracranial lesions, and can identify the presence or absence of associated abnormalities (see Fig. 4). Such associated abnormalities include callosal agenesis in the case of interhemispheric arachnoid cysts, parenchymal cysts in syndromes, and dorsal cysts seen in association with holoprosencephaly. At times, the cerebrospinal fluid (CSF) collections

seen in hydranencephaly may also be confused with a cystic mass.

Fetal MR imaging can also be used to image and characterize masses [71–74]. As with cystic collections, MR often can identify if masses are extracranial, intracranial-extra-axial, or intra-axial. It can also differentiate cystic from solid and mixed lesions, thus helping to develop a differential diagnosis (Fig. 10). The differential of fetal intracranial tumors includes teratomas, choroid plexus papillomas, gangliogliomas, astrocytomas, and glioblastomas, and primitive neuroectodermal tumors [75,76].

MR imaging may also be useful in the evaluation of fetuses suspected of having tuberous sclerosis following the discovery of a cardiac mass suspicious for a rhabdomyoma on prenatal imaging [77]. Although MR is much more sensitive than ultrasound for detecting subependymal

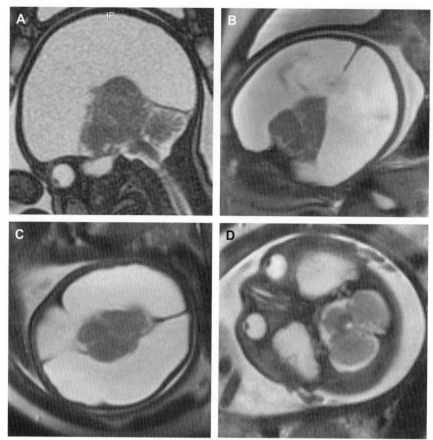

Fig. 18. Hydranencephaly: prenatal brain MR images (*A*, *B*, *C*, *D*). Sagittal true FISP (*A*) and coronal (*B*) and axial (*C*, *D*) T2-weighted HASTE images at 32 weeks of gestation demonstrate macrocephaly. The cerebral hemispheres are absent completely and are replaced by CSF fluid collections. A midline falx is present (*C*). The brainstem and cerebellum are normally developed (*D*).

nodules or tubers in fetuses with tuberous sclerosis, the absence of visualized lesions on MR images does not rule out the diagnosis. Hamartomas and tubers demonstrate high signal intensity on T1-weighted images and low signal intensity on T2-weighted sequences [77,78]. A case of a fetal subependymal giant cell astrocytoma has also been reported [79].

The extent of extracranial masses, their effect on adjacent structures, and their possible intracranial extension can be evaluated using MR. Images can demonstrate if lesions are cystic, solid, or mixed in nature, and this, together with information on the location and vascularity of the lesion, often can help determine the diagnosis (Figs. 11 and 12). Such masses include encephaloceles, teratomas, and rhabdomyosarcomas, and hemangiomas, lymphangiomas, and other soft-tissue masses [80].

When lesions extend into the neck, they may cause compression or obstruction of the airway. If the compression is severe, intensive maternal-fetal monitoring is required during delivery and an ex utero intrapartum treatment (EXIT) procedure may be needed. During this procedure, the infant is delivered by caesarian section; fetoplacental circulation is maintained while the airway is secured [80,81].

Fetal MR imaging can be useful in the evaluation and differentiation of chest lesions when the question of a mass in this region is raised by prenatal ultrasound [82–85]. The differential diagnosis includes congenital cystic adenomatoid malformation (CCAM), sequestration, and congenital diaphragmatic hernia [82]. T2-weighted HASTE images identify the location and extent of mass lesions readily and may identify the cystic nature of CCAMs (Figs. 13 and 14). The authors have found T2-weighted true FISP images to be useful particularly in demonstrating the position of the liver in patients' chest lesions; this information helps identify the presence of congenital diaphragmatic hernias and also gives prognostic information, because those cases with herniation of the liver above the diaphragm have a worse prognosis [86]. T1-weighted imaging may also be useful because it may show the presence of high T1 signal intensity, meconium-filled bowel loops extending into the chest, thus helping to distinguish diaphragmatic hernias from CCAMs containing large cysts (Fig. 15) [24]. Fetal MR imaging is able to identify the amount of adjacent lung present as well, information that may be useful in predicting future prognosis [87,88]. On serial studies, CCAMs may be seen to decrease in size as the fetus matures [89].

Multiplanar fetal MR imaging can also identify abdominal and pelvic masses, and can help to create a differential diagnosis by characterizing the lesion (solid, cystic, mixed, or hemorrhagic) and defining its organ of origin (Fig. 16) [90–92]. Often, in this way, liver tumors (hemangioendotheliomas, hepatoblastomas, metastatic neuroblastomas, and mesenchymal hamartomas), adrenal lesions (neuroblastomas and hematomas), renal lesions (hydronephrosis, renal cystic lesions, and tumors such as mesoblastic nephroma and, rarely, Wilms tumor), and retroperitoneal lesions (teratoma and infradiaphragmatic extralobar pulmonary sequestration) can be differentiated [93].

Is here a destructive brain lesion or the presence of hemorrhage?

Areas of hemorrhage may be seen on fetal MR studies and usually are identified as areas of high signal intensity on T1-weighted images and low signal intensity on T2-weighted images (Fig. 17) [24,94–96]. They may be identified better on gradient-echo T2*-weighted images [97]. Hemorrhage may occur following hypoxic/ischemic injury or bleeding of an underlying vascular malformation; in fetuses with clotting abnormalities; or secondary to maternal trauma, infection, or drug use. Spontaneous resolution of prenatally diagnosed intracranial hemorrhages has also been reported [98]. The literature reports several instances of

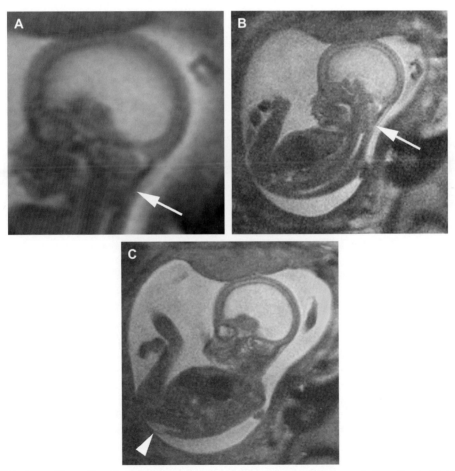

Fig. 19. Chiari II malformation. Sagittal (*A*) midline true FISP image at 20 weeks gestation demonstrates a small posterior fossa and inferior herniation of the cerebellar tonsils (*arrow*). Additional sagittal (*B, C*) T2-weighted HASTE images show the tonsillar herniation (*arrow*) and a posterior lumbar myelomeningocele (*arrowhead*).

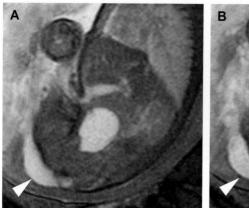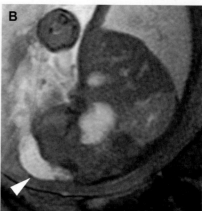

Fig. 20. Sacral teratoma. Sagittal (*A, B*) true FISP images at 30 weeks gestation demonstrate a multiloculated elongated cystic perineal mass (*arrowhead*) with no definitive connection to the spinal canal.

prenatally diagnosed vascular malformations, including vein of Galen aneurysms [99–101], dural sinus malformations, and pial arteriovenous fistulas [102].

Nonhemorrhagic ischemic lesions also may be seen on fetal MR imaging studies [97,103–105]; their causes may be of placental, fetal (infection, anasarca), or maternal (hypovolemic shock, hypoxia, abdominal trauma, hypotension, drug use) origin [97]. Monochorionic twins and fetuses with congenital infections have an increased risk of their occurrence [66]. Lesions may involve the cortex (delay of cortical development, polymicrogyria, laminar necrosis), the white matter (periventricular leukomalacia, calcification), or both (hydranencephaly) (Fig. 18). Areas of laminar necrosis and periventricular leukomalacia demonstrate high signal intensity on T1-weighted images and low signal intensity on T2-weighted images; areas of cavitation and gliosis show high T2 signal intensity [97]. Smaller lesions may be identified as areas of high T2 signal intensity in the periventricular regions, or as focal defects in the gray matter. In the future, diffusion-weighted imaging may play a greater role in the evaluation of this group of patients.

Is spinal dysraphism present?

MR can be used to image the spinal cord and spinal canal directly, when fetal ultrasound demonstrates or raises the question of spinal dysraphism. The literature reports some disagreement regarding the value of fetal MR over prenatal ultrasound (Fig. 19) [13,106–108]. Most investigators feel that fetal MR is a complementary modality, and although prenatal ultrasound may be superior to MR at detecting the level of the abnormality, identifying the presence of bony lesions, and giving

information on the lower extremities, MR shows the anatomy of the spinal cord better and defines any associated brain lesions [14,66]. It may therefore be useful in the demonstration of both spina bifida aperta and occult spinal dysraphism, and it has been found to be useful in the evaluation of fetuses with meningoceles, myeloceles, meningomyeloceles, meningocystoceles, diastematomyelia, caudal regression, and segmental spinal dysgenesis [14,66,109].

In fetuses with Chiari II malformations, fetal MR can also visualize clearly the presence of ventriculomegaly, the small posterior fossa, and herniation of the cerebellar tonsils (see Fig. 19) [4,14,66]. It may also be useful in the evaluation of spinal and presacral tumors, including teratomas, dermoids and epidermoids, and hamartomas (Fig. 20) [110].

A multicenter national trial is underway to evaluate the role of fetal surgery in cases of myelomeningocele [111]. If the results of this study indicate improved outcome in affected fetuses following surgery, then MR preoperative mapping will become routine in this group of patients [66]. Factors that support inclusion in the study include the presence of a low myelomeningocele, demonstration of normal leg motion, and absence of club feet and associated congenital anomalies [4]. Follow-up imaging after surgery frequently shows the reappearance of the CSF spaces around the posterior fossa structures.

Increased risk of anomalies being present

In some instances, fetal MR may be requested when there is an increased likelihood that an anomaly may be present. Such instances occur when a previous child has had a congenital anomaly or the family has a history of a genetic disorder, in cases of monochorionic twinning because of the increased risk of problems resulting from twin-twin trans- fusions and co-twin demise, and when there is a his- tory of a maternal illness (infection or cardiac event.) In these situations, confirmation that no abnormality is present can be extremely reassuring to parents.

Summary

Fetal MR imaging plays a complementary role to prenatal ultrasound in the evaluation of the fetus with suspected abnormalities. MR imaging's role includes confirming or excluding possible lesions, defining their full extent, aiding in their character- ization, and demonstrating other associated abnor- malities. As newer techniques such as diffusion imaging, MR spectroscopy, and functional studies are used more widely, it is hoped that additional in- formation will be made available by this modality to physicians evaluating and taking care of fetuses.

References

[1] Sonigo PC, Rypens FF, Carteret M, et al. MR im- aging of fetal cerebral anomalies. Pediatr Radiol 1998;28(4):212–22.

[2] Levine D. Fetal magnetic resonance imaging. J Matern Fetal Neonatal Med 2004;15:85–94.

[3] Golja AM, Estroff JA, Robertson RL. Fetal imag- ing of central nervous system abnormalities. Neuroimaging Clin N Am 2004;14:293–306.

[4] Zimmerman RA, Bilaniuk L. Magnetic reso- nance evaluation of fetal ventriculomegaly- associated congenital malformations and lesions. Semin Fetal Neonatal Med 2005;10: 429–43.

[5] Glenn O. Fetal central nervous system MR imag- ing. Neuroimaging clin N Am 2006;16:1–17.

[6] Gressens P, Luton D. Fetal MRI: obstetrical and neurological perspectives. Pediatr Radiol 2004; 34(9):682–4.

[7] Coakley FV, Hricak H, Filly RA, et al. Complex fetal disorders: effect of MR imaging on man- agement—preliminary clinical experience. Radi- ology 1999;213:691–6.

[8] Levine D, Barnes PD, Madsen JR, et al. Central nervous system abnormalities assessed with prenatal magnetic resonance imaging. Obstet Gynecol 1999;94:1011–9.

[9] Simon EM, Goldstein RB, Coakley FV, et al. Fast MR imaging of fetal CNS anomalies in utero. AJNR Am J Neuroradiol 2000;21:1688–98.

[10] Whitby EH, Paley MNJ, Sprigg A, et al. Com- parison of ultrasound and magnetic resonance imaging in 100 singleton pregnancies with sus- pected brain abnormalities. BJOG 2004;111: 784–92.

[11] Blaicher W, Prayer D, Mittermayer C, et al. The clinical impact of magnetic resonance imaging

in fetuses with central nervous system anoma- lies on ultrasound scan. Ultraschall Med 2005; 26:29–35.

[12] Frates M, Kumar A, Benson C, et al. Fetal anom- alies: comparison of MR imaging and US for diagnosis. Radiology 2004;232:398–404.

[13] Griffiths PD, Widjaja E, Paley MN, et al. Imag- ing the fetal spine using in utero MR: diagnostic accuracy and impact on management. Pediatr Radiol 2006;36(9):927–33.

[14] Simon EM. MRI of the fetal spine. Pediatr Radiol 2004;34(9):712–9.

[15] De Wilde JP, Rivers AW, Price DL. A review of the current use of magnetic resonance imaging in pregnancy and safety implications for the fetus. Prog Biophys Mol Biol 2005;87:335–53.

[16] Baker P, Johnson I, Harvey R, et al. A three-year follow-up on children imaged in utero with echo-planar magnetic resonance. Am J Obstet Gynecol 1994;170:32–3.

[17] Glover P, Hykin J, Gowland PA, et al. An as- sessment of the intrauterine sound intensity level during obstetric echo-planar magnetic resonance imaging. Br J Radiol 1995;68: 1090–4.

[18] Clements H, Duncan KR, Fielding K, et al. Infants exposed to MRI in utero have a normal paediatric assessment at 9 months of age. Fr J Radiol 2000;73:190–4.

[19] Kok RD, de Vries MM, Heerschap A, et al. Ab- sence of harmful effects of magnetic resonance exposure at 1.5 T in utero during the third tri- mester of pregnancy: a follow-up study. Magn Reson Imaging 2004;22:851–4.

[20] Kanal E, Gillen J, Evans JA, et al. Survey of re- productive health among female MR workers. Radiology 1993;187:395–9.

[21] Myers C, Duncan KR, Gowland PA, et al. Failure to detect intrauterine growth restriction follow- ing in utero exposure to MRI. Br J Radiol 1998; 71:549–51.

[22] Kanal E, Borgstede JP, Barkovich AJ, et al. Ameri- can college of radiology white paper on MR safety. AJR Am J Roentgenol 2002;178:1335–47.

[23] Chung HW, Chen CY, Zimmerman R, et al. T2- Weighted fast MR imaging with true FISP versus HASTE: comparative efficacy in the evaluation of normal fetal brain maturation. AJR Am J Roentgenol 2000;175(5):1375–80.

[24] Zizka J, Elias P, Hodik K, et al. Liver, meconium, haemorrhage: the value of T1-weighted images in fetal MRI. Pediatr Radiol 2006;36:792–801.

[25] Prayer D, Brugger PC, Prayer L. Fetal MRI: tech- niques and protocols. Pediatr Radiol 2004;34: 685–93.

[26] Glen O, Barkovich AJ. Magnetic resonance im- aging of the fetal brain and spine: an increas- ingly important tool in prenatal diagnosis, part I. AJNR Am J Neuroradiol 2006;27(8): 1604–11.

[27] Garel C. New advances in fetal MR neuroimag- ing. Pediatr Radiol 2006;36:621–5.

[28] Agid R, Lieberman S, Nadjari M, et al. Prenatal MR diffusion-weighted imaging in a fetus with hemimegalencephaly. Pediatr Radiol 2006;36: 138–40.

[29] Guo W, Ono S, Oi S, et al. Dynamic motion analysis of fetuses with central nervous system disorders by cine magnetic resonance imaging using fast imaging employing steady-state acquisition and parallel imaging: a preliminary result. J Neurosur 2006;105:94–100.

[30] Girard N, Gouny S, Viola A, et al. Assessment of normal fetal brain maturation in utero by proton magnetic resonance spectroscopy. Magn Reson Med 2006;56:768–75.

[31] Heerschap A, Kok RD, van den Berg PP. Antenatal proton MR spectroscopy of the human brain in vivo. Childs Nerv Syst 2003;19:418–21.

[32] Fenton BW, Lin CS, Macedonia C, et al. The fetus at term: in utero volume-selected proton MR spectroscopy with a breath-hold technique—a feasibility study. Radiology 2001;219: 563–6.

[33] Kok RD, van den Berg AJ, Heerschap A, et al. Metabolic information from the human fetal brain obtained with proton magnetic resonance spectroscopy. Am J Obstet Gynecol 2001;185:1011–5.

[34] Roelants-van Rijn AM, Groenendaal F, Stoutenbeek P, et al. Lactate in the foetal brain: detection and implications. Acta Paediatr 2004; 93:937–40.

[35] Kok RD, van den Berg PP, van den Berg AJ, et al. Maturation of the human fetal brain as observed by H MR spectroscopy. Magn Reson Med 2002;48:611–6.

[36] Girard N, Raybaud C, Poncet M. In vivo MR study of brain maturation in normal fetuses. AJNR Am J Neuroradiol; 1995;16:407–13.

[37] Brisse H, Fallet C, Sebag G, et al. Supratentorial parenchyma in the developing fetal brain: in vivo MR study with histologic comparison. AJNR Am J Neuroradiol 1997;18:1491–7.

[38] Garel C, Chantrel E, Brisse H, et al. Fetal cerebral cortex: normal gestational landmarks identified using prenatal MR imaging. AJNR Am J Neuroradiol 2001;22:184–9.

[39] Garel C, Chantrel E, Elmaleh M, et al. Fetal MRI: normal gestational landmarks for cerebral biometry, gyration and myelination. Childs Nerv Syst 2003;19:422–5.

[40] Levine D, Barnes PD. Cortical maturation in normal and abnormal fetuses as assessed with prenatal MR imaging. Radiology 1999;210:751–8.

[41] Girard N, Raybaud C. In vivo MRI of fetal brain cellular migration. J Comput Assist Tomogr 1992;16:265–7.

[42] Fogliarini C, Chaumoitre K, Chapon F, et al. Assessment of cortical maturation with prenatal MRI. Part I: normal cortical maturation. Eur Radiol 2005;15:1671–85.

[43] Triulzi F, Parazzini C, Righini A. MRI of fetal and neonatal cerebellar development. Semin Fetal Neonatal Med 2005;10:411–20.

[44] Adamsbaum C, Moutard M, Andre C, et al. MRI of the fetal posterior fossa. Pediatr Radiol 2005; 34:124–40.

[45] Garel C, editor. MRI of the fetal brain. Normal development and cerebral pathologies. Berlin: Springer; 2004. p. 35–114.

[46] Chen S, Simon E, Haselgrove J, et al. Fetal posterior fossa volume: assessment with MR imaging. Radiology 2006;238:997–1003.

[47] Garel C, Alberti C. Coronal measurement of the fetal lateral ventricles: comparison between ultrasonography and magnetic resonance imaging. Ultrasound obstet gynecol 2006;27:23–7.

[48] Grossman R, Hoffman C, Mardor Y, et al. Quantitative MRI measurements of human fetal brain development in utero. Neuroimage 2006; 33:463–70.

[49] Watanabe Y, Abe S, Takagi K, et al. Evolution of subarachnoid space in normal fetuses using magnetic resonance imaging. Prenat Diagn 2005;25:1217–22.

[50] Breeze AC, Alexander PM, Murdoch EM, et al. Obstetric and neonatal outcomes in severe fetal ventriculomegaly. Prenat Diagn 2007;27(2): 124–9.

[51] Breeze AC, Dey P, Lees C, et al. Obstetric and neonatal outcomes in apparently isolated mild fetal ventriculomegaly. J Perinat Med 2005;33: 236–40.

[52] Ouahba J, Luton D, Vuillard E, et al. Prenatal isolated mild ventriculomegaly: outcome in 167 cases. BJOG 2006;113:1072–9.

[53] Valsky D, Ben-Sira L, Porat S, et al. The role of magnetic resonance imaging in the evaluation of isolated mild ventriculomegaly. J Ultrasound Med 2004;23:519–23.

[54] Salomon LJ, Ouahba J, Delezoide A-L, et al. Third-trimester fetal MRI in isolated 10- to 12-mm ventriculomegaly: is it worth it? BJOG 2006;113:942–7.

[55] Glenn O, Goldstein R, Li K, et al. Fetal magnetic resonance imaging in the evaluation of fetuses referred for sonographically suspected abnormalities of the corpus callosum. J Ultrasound Med 2005;24:791–804.

[56] Ickowitz V, Eurin D, Rypens F, et al. Prenatal diagnosis and postnatal follow-up of pericallosal lipoma: report of seven new cases. AJNR Am J Neuroradiol 2001;22:767–72.

[57] Volpe P, Paladini D, Resta M, et al. Characteristics, associations and outcome of partial agenesis of the corpus callosum in the fetus. Ultrasound Obstet Gynecol 2006;27: 509–16.

[58] Barkovich AJ, Norman D. Anomalies of the corpus callosum: correlation with further anomalies of the brain. AJNR Am J Neuroradiol 1988;151(1):171–9.

[59] Toma P, Costa A, Magnano GM, et al. Holoprosencephaly: prenatal diagnosis by sonography and magnetic resonance imaging. Prenat Diagn 1990;10(7):429–36.

[60] Wong AM, Bilaniuk LT, Ng KK, et al. Lobar holoprosencephaly: prenatal MR diagnosis with postnatal MR correlation. Prenat Diagn 2005;25(4):296–9.

[61] Pulizer S, Simon E, Crombleholme T, et al. Prenatal MR findings of the middle interhemispheric variant of holoprosencephaly. AJNR Am J Neuroradiol 2004;25:1034–6.

[62] Fogliarini C, Chaumoitre K, Chapon F, et al. Assessment of cortical maturation with prenatal MRI: part II: abnormalities of cortical maturation. Eur Radiol 2005;15:1781–9.

[63] Rubod C, Robert Y, Tillouche N, et al. Role of fetal ultrasound and magnetic resonance imaging in the prenatal diagnosis of migration disorders. Prenat Diagn 2005;25:1181–7.

[64] Fong KW, Ghai S, Toi A, et al. Prenatal ultrasound findings of lissencephaly associated with Miller-Dieker syndrome and comparison with pre- and postnatal magnetic resonance imaging. Ultrasound Obstet Gynecol 2004;24:716–23.

[65] Mochel F, Grebille AG, Benachi A, et al. Contribution of fetal MR imaging in the prenatal diagnosis of Zellweger syndrome. AJNR Am J Neuroradiol 2006;27:333–6.

[66] Glenn OA, Barkovich J. Magnetic resonance imaging of the fetal brain and spine: an increasingly important tool in prenatal diagnosis: part 2. AJNR Am J Neuroradiol 2006;27:1807–14.

[67] Limperopoulos C, Robertson R, Estroff J, et al. Diagnosis of inferior vermian hypoplasia by fetal magnetic resonance imaging: potential pitfalls and neurodevelopmental outcome. Am J Obstet Gynecol 2006;194:1070–6.

[68] Napolitano M, Righini A, Zirpoli S, et al. Prenatal magnetic resonance imaging of rhombencephalosynapsis and associated brain anomalies: report of 3 cases. J Comput Assist Tomogr 2004;28:762–5.

[69] Smith AS, Levine D, Barnes P, et al. Magnetic resonance imaging of the kinked fetal brain stem: a sign of severe dysgenesis. J Ultrasound Med 2005;24:1697–709.

[70] Fluss J, Blaser S, Chitayat D, et al. Molar tooth sign in fetal brain magnetic resonance imaging leading to the prenatal diagnosis of Joubert syndrome and related disorders. J Child Neurol 2006;21:320–4.

[71] Doherty D, Glass I, Siebert J, et al. Prenatal diagnosis in pregnancies at risk for Joubert syndrome by ultrasound and MRI. Prenat Diagn 2005;25:442–7.

[72] Chuang YM, Guo WY, Ho DM, et al. Skew ocular deviation: a catastrophic sign on MRI of fetal glioblastoma. Childs Nerv Syst 2003;19(5–6):371–5.

[73] Muhonen MG, Bierman JS, Hussain NS, et al. Giant intracranial teratoma and lack of cortical development in a fetus. Case report. J Neurosurg 2005;103(Suppl 2):180–3.

[74] Marden FA, Wippold FJ 2nd, Perry A. Fast magnetic resonance imaging in steady-state precession (true FISP) in the prenatal diagnosis of a congenital brain teratoma. J Comput Assist Tomogr 2003;27(3):427–30.

[75] Isaacs H Jr II. Perinatal brain tumors: a review of 250 cases. Pediatr Neurol 2002;27(5):333–42.

[76] Woodward PJ, Sohaey R, Kennedy A, et al. From the archives of the AFIP: a comprehensive review of fetal tumors with pathologic correlation. Radiographics 2005;25(1):215–42.

[77] Chen CP, Liu YP, Huang JK, et al. Contribution of ultrafast magnetic resonance imaging in prenatal diagnosis of sonographically undetected cerebral tuberous sclerosis associated with cardiac rhabdomyomas. Prenat Diagn 2005;25:523–4.

[78] Levine D, Barnes P, Korf B, et al. Tuberous sclerosis in the fetus: second-trimester diagnosis of subependymal tubers with ultrafast MR imaging. Am J Radiol 2000;175:1067–9.

[79] Hussain N, Curran A, Pilling D, et al. Congenital subependymal giant cell astrocytoma diagnosed on fetal MRI. Arch Dis Child 2006;91(6):520.

[80] Robson CD, Barnewolt C. MR imaging of fetal head and neck anomalies. Neuroimaging Clin N Am 2004;14:273–91.

[81] Hubbard AM. Magnetic resonance imaging of fetal thoracic abnormalities. Top Magn Reson Imaging 2001;12(1):18–24.

[82] Hubbard AM, Simon EM. Fetal imaging. Magn Reson Imaging Clin N Am 2002;10(2):389–408.

[83] Levine D, Barnewolt CE, Mehta TS, et al. Fetal thoracic abnormalities. MR Imaging Radiol 2003;228:379–88.

[84] Johnson AM, Hubbard AM. Congenital abnormalities of the fetal/neonatal chest. Semin Roentgenol 2004;39(2):197–214.

[85] Levine D. Fetal magnetic resonance imaging. J Maternal-Fetal Neonatal Med 2004;15:85.

[86] Kitano Y, Nakagawa S, Kuroda T, et al. Liver position in fetal congenital diaphragmatic hernia retains a prognostic value in the era of lung-protective strategy. J Pediatr Surg 2005;40:1827–32.

[87] Gorincour G, Bouvenot J, Mourot MG, et al. Prenatal prognosis of congenital diaphragmatic hernia using magnetic resonance imaging measurement of fetal lung volume. Ultrasound Obstet Gynecol 2005;26:738–44.

[88] Kawamura M, Itoh H, Yamada S, et al. Spontaneous regression of congenital cystic adenomatoid malformation of the lung: longitudinal examinations by magnetic resonance imaging. Congenit Anom (Kyoto) 2005;45:157–60.

[89] Williams G, Coakley FV, Qayyum A, et al. Fetal relative lung volume: quantification by using prenatal MR imaging lung volumetry. Radiology 2004;233:457–62.

[90] Martin C, Darnell A, Duran C, et al. Magnetic resonance imaging of the intrauterine fetal genitourinary tract: normal anatomy and pathology. Abdom Imaging 2004;29:286–302.

[91] Liu YP, Cheng SJ, Shih SL, et al. Autosomal recessive polycystic kidney disease: appearance on fetal MRI. Pediatr Radiol 2006;36:169.

[92] Aslan H, Ozseker B, Gul A. Prenatal sonographic and magnetic resonance imaging diagnosis of cystic neuroblastoma. Ultrasound Obstet Gynecol 2004;24:693–4.

[93] Dietrich RB. Pediatric body MRI. In: Stark DD, Bradley WG, editors. Magnetic resonance imaging. 3rd edition. St. Louis (MO): CV Mosby Co., Inc.; 1998. p. 658–72.

[94] Trop I, Levine D. Hemorrhage during pregnancy: sonography and MR imaging. Am J Radiol 2001;176:607–15.

[95] Gorincour G, Rypens F, Lapierre C, et al. Fetal magnetic resonance imaging in the prenatal diagnosis of cerebellar hemorrhage. Ultrasound Obstet Gynecol 2006;27:78–80.

[96] Morioka T, Hashiguchi K, Nagata S, et al. Fetal germinal matrix and intraventricular hemorrhage. Pediatr Neurosurg 2006;42:354–61.

[97] Garel C, Delezoide AL, Elmaleh Berges M, et al. Contribution of fetal MR imaging in the evaluation of cerebral ischemic lesions. AJNR Am J Neuroradiol 2004;25:1563–8.

[98] Barrozzino T, Sgro M, Toi A, et al. Fetal bilateral subdural haemorrhages. Prenatal diagnosis and spontaneous resolution by time of delivery. Prenat Diagn 1998;18(5):496–503.

[99] Campi A, Scotti G, Filippi M, et al. Antenatal diagnosis of vein of Galen aneurismal malformation: MR study of fetal brain and postnatal follow-up. Neuroradiology 1996;38(1):87–90.

[100] Kurihara N, Tokieda K, Ikeda K, et al. Prenatal MR findings in a case of aneurysm of the vein of Galen. Pediatr Radiol 2001;31(3):160–2.

[101] Messori A, Polonara G, Salvolini U. Prenatal diagnosis of a vein of Galen aneurismal malformation with fetal MR imaging study. AJNR Am J Neuroradiol 2003;24:1923–5.

[102] Garel C, Azarian M, Lasjaunias P, et al. Pial arteriovenous fistulas: dilemmas in prenatal diagnosis, counseling and postnatal treatment. Report of three cases. Ultrasound Obstet Gynecol 2005;26:293–6.

[103] de Laveaucoupet J, Audibert F, Guis F, et al. Fetal magnetic resonance imaging (MRI) of ischemic brain injury. Prenat Diagn 2001;21(9):729–36.

[104] Brunel H, Girard N, Confort-Gouny S, et al. Fetal brain injury. J Neuroradiol 2004;31(2): 123–37.

[105] Girard N, Chaumoitre K, Confort-Gouny S, et al. Magnetic resonance imaging and the detection of fetal brain anomalies, injury, and physiologic adaptations. Curr Opin Obstet Gynecol 2006;18:164–76.

[106] von Koch C, Glenn OA, Goldstein RB, et al. Fetal magnetic resonance imaging enhances detection of spinal cord anomalies in patients with sonographically detected bony anomalies of the spine. J Ultrasound Med 2005;24: 781–9.

[107] Appasamy M, Roberts D, Pilling D, et al. Antenatal ultrasound and magnetic resonance imaging in localizing the level of lesion in spina bifida and correlation with postnatal outcome. Ultrasound Obstet Gynecol 2006;27:530–6.

[108] Aaronson OS, Hernanz-Schulman M, Bruner JP, et al. Myelomeningocele: prenatal evaluation—comparison between transabdominal US and MR imaging. Radiology 2003;224:839–43.

[109] Mangels KJ, Tulipan N, Tsao LY, et al. Fetal MRI in the evaluation of intrauterine myelomeningocele. Pediatr Neurosurg 2000;32(2):124–31.

[110] Danzer E, Hubbard AM, Hedrick HL, et al. Diagnosis and characterization of fetal sacrococcygeal teratoma with prenatal MRI. Am J Roentgenol 2006;187:W350–6.

[111] Tulipan N. Intrauterine closure of myelomeningocele: an update. Neurosurg Focus 2004;16(2):E2.

ELSEVIER
SAUNDERS

MAGNETIC
RESONANCE
IMAGING CLINICS

Magn Reson Imaging Clin N Am 14 (2007) 523–535

MR Imaging Evaluation of the Pelvic Floor for the Assessment of Vaginal Prolapse and Urinary Incontinence

Diego R. Martin, MD, PhD[a],*, Khalil Salman, MD[b],
Chester C. Wilmot, MD[c], Niall T.M. Galloway, MD[c,d]

Female stress urinary incontinence (SUI) affects a large proportion of the female population. The role of MR imaging to date has been largely descriptive of the more conspicuous anatomic relations of the bony pelvis and soft tissues. Unfortunately, these approaches have not identified the important structural support mechanisms critical for therapeutic intervention and have not been useful from the perspective of planning surgical repairs. In this review, the authors report the identification of soft tissue structures, first identified on surgical anatomy and then correlated with the MR imaging findings, to show the soft tissue structures of pelvic support anatomy. These structures are critical to understanding the mechanisms of vaginal prolapse and for planning effective surgical repair.

Review of the clinical problem

Epidemiology

Urinary incontinence is defined as "the complaint of any involuntary leakage of urine," as recently simplified by the International Continence Society. Of the estimated 19 million North American adults who have urinary incontinence, 80% are women [1]. It is one of the most prevalent chronic diseases,

[a] Department of Radiology, Emory University School of Medicine, Emory University Hospital, Building A, AT622, 1365 Clifton Road, NE, Atlanta, GA 30322, USA
[b] Department of Radiology, Emory University School of Medicine, Atlanta, GA, USA
[c] Department of Urology, Emory University School of Medicine, 1365 Clifton Road, NE, Atlanta, GA 30322, USA
[d] Emory Continence Center, Emory University School of Medicine, Atlanta, GA 30322, USA
* Corresponding author.
E-mail address: diego_martin@emoryhealthcare.org (D.R. Martin).

1064-9689/07/$ – see front matter © 2007 Elsevier Inc. All rights reserved.
mri.theclinics.com

doi:10.1016/j.mric.2007.01.004

affecting from 15% to 50% of women of all ages, and is associated with a significant impact on quality of life and increasing financial cost. Many women fail to seek treatment because of embarrassment or the belief that incontinence is inevitable. Most urinary incontinence occurs through the urethra and is subclassified into SUI, urge urinary incontinence (UUI), and mixed urinary incontinence (MUI).

SUI is the loss of urine associated with events that increase intra-abdominal pressure and, as a result, increase pressure in the urinary bladder. Events that might provoke SUI include coughing, sneezing, lifting, bending, or exercise. It is the most common type of incontinence affecting younger women and is typically associated with some degree of urethral hypermobility and anterior vaginal wall prolapse. The most common predisposing factors include vaginal deliveries, pelvic surgery (eg, hysterectomy), accidental trauma, or radiation.

Urinary incontinence also commonly coexists with symptomatic disorders of pelvic prolapse, and at least 40% to 60% of women with SUI require a concurrent procedure for pelvic organ prolapse (POP) at the time of incontinence surgery. When the tissues of the pelvic floor become overstretched, weakened, or disrupted, that disturbance of normal pelvic support anatomy results in displacement of the internal organs, including the bladder, urethra, vagina, cervix, and uterus. These organs can prolapse into the genitourinary hiatus, and this is a common cause of SUI.

UUI is associated with a strong desire to urinate, with little warning or time to reach a bathroom. It is mostly associated with causes of an overactive bladder. UUI typically occurs in middle- or advanced-age patients, but it can occur at a younger age as well. The causes for UUI are not as fully characterized. Aging itself may not be the cause but is a risk factor. Causes of bladder irritation may be associated with UUI and include bladder infection, stones, or tumor. Less commonly, neurologic disease may cause or contribute to bladder dysfunction and may manifest in association with underlying neurologic disorders, such as multiple sclerosis or spinal cord diseases, including tumors.

Some women experience SUI and UUI at different times or under different circumstances; this condition is referred to as MUI. The causes of the two forms may or may not be related and should be evaluated separately.

Diagnosis and therapy

The type of incontinence is usually determined by the combination of history and physical examination. In a subset of patients, urodynamic testing may contribute to the assessment of urinary incontinence. Urodynamic testing measures pressure and volume within the bladder and flow or leakage from the urethra to determine patterns suggesting bladder or urethral dysfunction. Today, a standardized, reliable, and reproducible set of tools for fully evaluating pelvic support anatomy does not exist. Ideally, these would include tools that do not require high technology, allowing for more widespread adoption. Currently, the pelvic organ prolapse quantitation (POP-Q) score developed by the International Continence Society with the American Urogynecology Society of Gynecologic Surgeons is used and is determined by physical examination.

Treatment strategies include behavior modification to control urine output by controlling fluid intake and avoidance of dietary diuretics, such as caffeine. Pelvic floor therapy, including Kegel exercises, can increase pelvic muscle strength and endurance and has been shown to improve both types of urinary incontinence. Whether individuals experience incontinence or not, it has been suggested that all women should start doing Kegel exercises in their teenage years and continue throughout life.

Surgery remains the major form of therapy for SUI. Surgical repair may be highly successful and sometimes not only improves SUI but UUI. There remains controversy regarding procedures and definition of important anatomic relations and structures related to the mechanisms of pelvic floor instability and repair, however. Repair leading to therapeutic improvement does not necessarily require repair of all the disrupted tissues but only those that provide critical support in regard to continence. The lack of education and consensus on these relations can contribute to surgical causes of incontinence when a surgical procedure (eg, hysterectomy) may lead to inadvertent disruption of important support structures.

When performing surgery for incontinence, a comprehensive and anatomic approach intended for pelvic floor reconstruction is recommended [2]. Pelvic floor anatomy is complex, and pelvic floor defects may exist as a constellation of structural changes. These changes result in a variety of externally appreciable signs. Physical examination as the usual investigation alone is not always sufficient to characterize all the structural changes present. The goal of reconstructive surgery is to recreate the normal anatomy, and thereby restore function. To identify the critical structural changes present and restore normal anatomy, investigational modalities other than physical examination are needed.

Pelvic anatomy

Normal support

The pelvic floor consists of several components lying between the pelvic peritoneum and the vulvar skin. The viscera are actually part of the pelvic floor. Cranially to caudally, these structures are the peritoneum, the pelvic viscera, the endopelvic fascia, the levator ani muscle groups, and the perineal membrane and external genitalia. The support for all these structures comes from the connection to the bony pelvis and its attached muscles. The female pelvis is divided into anterior, middle, and posterior compartments. MR imaging allows for visualization of all three compartments. The vagina is attached laterally to the pelvic walls and acts as the single middle divider that determines the nature of any prolapse. The levator ani muscles form the bottom of the pelvis, and the endopelvic fascia forms a continuous sheet extending from the uterine artery cephalad to the point at which the vagina fuses with the levator ani muscles below. By clinical and surgical assessment, there are three general types of prolapse that can occur: (1) descent of the vaginal apex (apical prolapse), (2) protrusion of the anterior vaginal wall, or (3) protrusion of the posterior vaginal wall. The location of the prolapse determines whether a woman has a cystocele (anterior), rectocele (posterior), or vaginal vault prolapse (apical).

The uterus and cervix are attached to the pelvic side wall by the parametrium (composed of the cardinal and uterosacral ligaments). The parametrium courses downward over the upper vagina to the pelvic side wall, where it is called the paracolpium (level I support). The paracolpium provides support for the vaginal apex after hysterectomy. In the midportion of the vagina, the paracolpium attaches the vagina laterally and more directly to the pelvic side walls (level II support). This attachment stretches the vagina transversely between the bladder and rectum. The layer that supports the bladder is the pubocervical fascia, a combination of the anterior vaginal wall and its attachments to the pelvic wall. Similarly, the posterior vaginal wall and endopelvic fascia form a restraining layer that prevents the rectum from protruding forward (rectovaginal fascia). The distal vagina (level III support) is directly attached to the surrounding structures, fusing anteriorly with the urethra, posteriorly with the perineal body, and laterally with the levator ani muscles.

Damage to the upper suspensory fibers of the paracolpium causes uterine or vaginal vault prolapse. Damage to the level II and III supports of the vagina may result in the development of cystocele and rectocele. These defects occur in varying combinations and are responsible for the diversity of clinical problems.

The upper urethra and vesical neck are mobile structures, whereas the distal urethra remains in a fixed position. The anterior vaginal wall and urethra are intimately connected. The support structures for the midvagina are lateral to either side of the pelvis and are associated with a band of connective tissue that runs from the lower pubic bone to the ischial spine, which is known as the arcus tendineus fascia pelvis. These have been called the paravaginal attachments [3]. Loss of anterior vaginal support can occur because of lateral detachments (from the arcus tendineus) or as a central failure of the pubocervical fascia.

The urethral support mechanism holds the urethra in a position in which it can be compressed against the supporting hammock by rises in intra-abdominal pressure, a mechanism that may be required to prevent SUI. The multiple connections of the perineal body to the levator muscles and the pelvic walls prevent a low rectocele. Defects in the support at this level often occur from birth trauma.

Imaging can be useful to help confirm the clinically suspected prolapse, distinguish the prolapsing organ, and identify unsuspected defects in pelvic floor support.

Utility of pelvic MR imaging

Introduction

MR imaging has led to a breakthrough in the evaluation of pelvic floor disorders. Although it is not indicated in the routine evaluation of patients with uncomplicated primary urinary incontinence or POP [4], it has been used as a research tool for evaluation of the pelvic floor for more than a decade [5,6] and is now routinely used in several centers for preoperative planning of pelvic floor repairs. Early studies were limited by long scan times and poor resolution. MR imaging is the modality of choice for visualizing soft tissue structures, such as the viscera, pelvic musculature, and fascial investments, that comprise the pelvic support. MR imaging is noninvasive, involves no ionizing radiation, and results in superior cross-sectional depiction of pelvic anatomy. MR imaging has largely replaced other imaging modalities, such as ultrasound, colpocystodefecography (CCD), and voiding cystourethrography (VCUG), as the test of choice in evaluating the pelvic floor. It is essential that radiologists involved in the care of these patients be knowledgeable about the rapidly emerging potential of MR imaging in addressing these problems.

Radiologists' historical view of pelvic floor instability

To date, all imaging literature has focused attention on the anatomic bony landmarks of the pelvis to describe relations to soft tissues or for evaluation of the skeletal morphology in regard to risk factors for the development of SUI. MR imaging has been beneficial in this work to provide optimal visualization of the pelvic soft tissues. Although relations have been demonstrated, there has been little correlation between MR imaging and the surgical anatomy and MR imaging has not been fully used for elucidation of the mechanical principles of physical signs and corrective surgery.

Female pelvimetry

Architectural differences have been evaluated in the bony pelvis comparing multiparous women with and without pelvic floor disruption. For example, Handa and colleagues [7] performed a case-control study on patients who had pelvic MR imaging. Fifty-nine female patients with records indicating urinary symptoms and pelvic floor dysfunction were compared with 39 patients without symptoms. Women with pelvic floor prolapse were shown to have a wider transverse inlet, wider intertuberous diameter, wider interspinous diameter, greater sacrococcygeal length, deeper sacral curvature, and narrower anteroposterior outlet. Association with a wider transverse inlet and a shorter obstetric conjugate difference were found to be statistically significant with odds ratios of 3.425 and 0.233, respectively.

Pelvic soft tissues

MR imaging has been applied to the evaluation of the pelvic soft tissues in normal asymptomatic nulliparous [8], and symptomatic multiparous patients [9,10]. The soft tissues that have been described and analyzed have concentrated primarily on the levator ani and puborectalis muscles and have also examined dimensions related to the urogenital hiatus and the urethral length and cross section. The relation between the pelvic soft tissues and the bony pelvis has largely relied on assessment of the position of the urethra, vagina, and the rectum in relation to the pubococcygeal line (PCL) (Fig. 1). Dynamic MR imaging has been performed in conjunction with defecography with description of the anatomic position of the rectum in relation to the PCL and in relation to the angulation of the proximal rectum as compared with the distal rectum. Normally, the proximal rectum is relatively horizontal and the distal rectum is relatively vertical (see Fig. 1).

Normal soft tissue structures on MR imaging

A systematic approach to evaluation of pelvic support was proposed by Chou and DeLancey [11] after evaluation of axial images from 50 nulliparous women. A grid-based system was developed depicting pelvic support structures and their distance from a common landmark (the caudal arcuate

pubic ligament). These results showed a consistent location of structures despite not accounting for pelvic asymmetry or pelvic. There seems to be a wide inherent variability in normal pelvic support structures, however. Tunn and colleagues [8] evaluated 20 nulliparous women with 1.5-T axial images and found a wide degree of variability in levator ani area and thickness ranging from two- to threefold differences. There was no variability seen, however, for left versus right.

Anatomic changes on MR imaging related to prolapse

Deval and colleagues [12] showed that the sensitivity, specificity, and positive predictive value (PPV) of MR imaging were 70%, 100%, and 100% for the diagnosis of cystocele; 42%, 81%, and 60% for vaginal vault or uterine prolapse; 100%, 83%, and 75% for enterocele; and 87%, 72%, and 66% for rectocele, respectively. Other studies have reported lower figures and suggested the use of contrast medium to increase the diagnostic accuracy. Three-dimensional imaging has also been used to assess levator ani morphology and has shown that the levator ani morphologic features do not depend on the grade of prolapse and that not all women with pelvic prolapse have abnormal morphologic features [13].

Limitations

In summary, the bony and soft tissue relations to pelvic floor prolapse and incontinence have been largely descriptive of anatomic correlation with prolapse. These observations have frequently not considered the relation to the critical suspensory soft tissue structures defined as critical to symptomatic therapy, however. Soft tissue structures that have been the focus of many imaging studies, such as the levator ani, have not been found critical for surgical repair as determined by postsurgical symptomatic improvement.

Current and developing state of the art

From the perspective of surgical repair

Surgical pioneers recognized the importance of urethral hypermobility as a cause for SUI, and the first surgical procedures were directed simply to elevate and fix the urethra in a retropubic position with operations like the Marshall-Marchetti-Kranz (MMK) technique [14]. Many other procedures have followed, and they have offered incremental advances always creating some kind of compensating abnormality, attaching one structure to another or introducing an external agent, instead of trying to restore normal nulliparous anatomic relations. Vaginal surgeons accepted that bulges of the vaginal

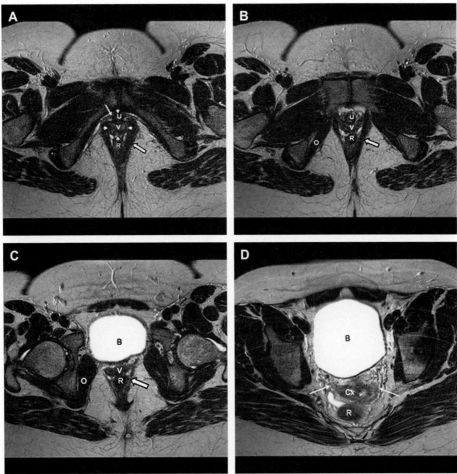

Fig. 1. Normal pelvis acquired on axial free-breathing fast spin echo (FSE) T2-weighted (*A–D*), coronal breath-hold single-shot T2-weighted (*E, F*), sagittal breath-hold single-shot T2-weighted (*G*) and free-breathing FSE T2-weighted (*H*) images. Axial images are obtained from inferior (*A*) to superior (*D*). (*A*) Image is obtained at the lower urogenital hiatus (*arrowheads*) demarcated anteriorly by the anterior urethra (U) and arcus tendineus (*thin arrow*), posteriorly by the rectum (R), and laterally by the lateral margins of the vagina (V) and inner aspect of the levator ani muscle (*thick arrow*). (*B*) Slightly more superiorly, the obturator internus (O) and levator ani (*thick arrow*) can be seen to attach anteriorly to the posterior inferior pubic bone. (*C*) More superiorly but still at the level of the midvagina, the levator ani is thinning and beginning to separate away from the lateral walls of the vagina. (*D*) Most superior axial slice is at the level of the external cervical os (Cx) and vaginal fornices (*arrows*). This level is above the levator ani, and the lateral pelvic walls are now visible. Note that the lateral vaginal fornices are well invested with connective tissue that envelopes the lateral walls of the vagina and connects with the lateral pelvic wall (*arrows*). On coronal imaging posteriorly (*E*) through the upper vagina and cervix and more anteriorly (*F*) through the midcervix, the investment of connective tissue (*arrows*) is shown. This connective tissue surrounds the cervix and upper vagina and extends superiorly along the pelvic side wall (*F, arrows*). The posterior and normally thin component of the levator ani is visualized (*F, arrowheads*), and the obturator internus is again identified (*F, O*). Sagittal cervix (*G*) and midline urethra (*H*) images show the pelvic organ anatomy in relation to the pelvic floor. The bony landmarks are easily identified on MR imaging and the pubococcygeal reference line (*dotted line; G, H*) is shown, extending from the undersurface of the symphysis pubis to the lower coccyx. The vaginal anterior (*black arrows, G*) and posterior (*white arrows, G*) walls are indicated, and the unique excellent soft tissue contrast delineation possible only on MR imaging is shown. In the midpelvis, note that the normal vagina is located well apposed to the posteroinferior wall of the bladder (B) and erect posterior to the urethra. The normal cervix is located high and posterior in the pelvis relative to the pubococcygeal reference line. In the posterior pelvis, note that the normal rectum is horizontal proximally and is angulated, becoming vertical distal to the anus. Technical note should be made of the excellent soft tissue detail that is achievable on free-breathing FSE (4-minute acquisition) and breath-hold single-shot (~20-second acquisition) sequences. In patients who may move excessively during the acquisition, however, the single-shot technique is much more resistant to image degradation.

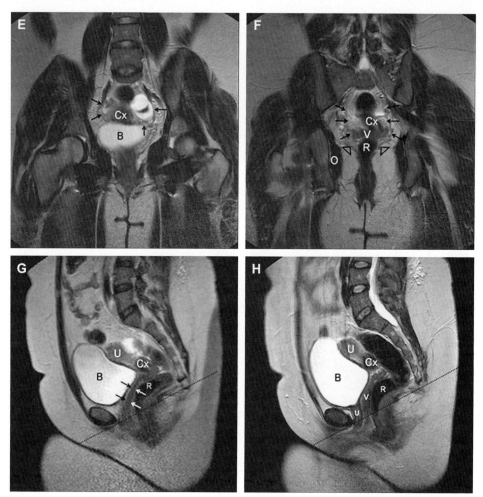

Fig. 1 (continued)

walls must be attributable to overstretching, thinning, and attenuation of the tissues. This led to procedures that were designed to plicate and shorten the vaginal tissues, such as anterior and posterior repairs.

Modern surgical anatomists like A.C. Richardson have defined the continuity of the endopelvic fascial attachments that make up the tensional network of normal pelvic support anatomy. When the pelvic support structures are intact, there are no vaginal bulges. When the pelvic support structures are intact, the urethra is not hypermobile, the bladder base is in normal anatomic position, and there is no POP. These observations have emphasized the importance of the less obvious pelvic support structures and clarified the patterns of defects and detachments that result in prolapse and SUI.

These observations have redefined the task of the pelvic surgeon, who can now recognize site-specific defects and detachments for repair and reconstruction. The paradigm of surgical repairs is changing from "sutures in the bulges" to targeted repair of site-specific defects and detachments to restore the integrity of the structural network that constitutes normal pelvic support anatomy. The defects can be repaired using surgical access that could be vaginal, abdominal, or minimally invasive. Richardson emphasized the importance of careful perineal examination before surgery and was often able to recognize or deduce the specific defects in a particular patient using physical examination alone.

One of the challenges has been how to image the pelvic support structures. It is important that surgeons are able to demonstrate accurately the presence of site-specific defects and detachments before surgery and also evaluate the postoperative changes and efficacy of surgical repairs. The authors have been interested in evaluating the role of high-definition MR imaging in the assessment of some of

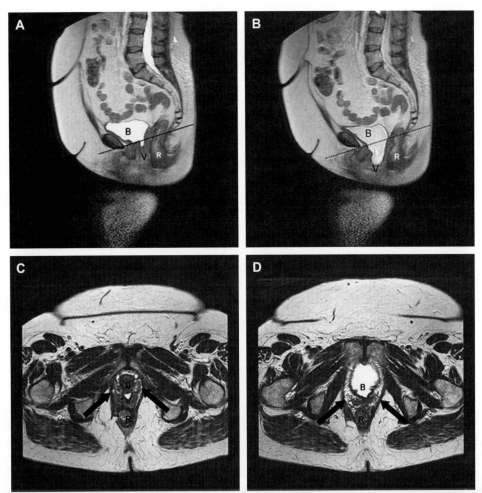

Fig. 2. Patient after hysterectomy with prolapse and bilateral disruption of the uterosacral ligaments. Sagittal SST2 dynamic imaging shows marked prolapse at rest (*A*) and exacerbated with stress (*B*). There is rectal, vaginal, and vesicular prolapse, with excursion below the pubo-coccygeal line (*A, B; dotted line*). The lower vagina (V)-urethral anterior attachments to the inferior aspect of the symphysis pubis remain intact, and this results in the vagina being pulled under the bladder (B) as the bladder falls through the pelvic floor and pushes onto the anterior wall of the vagina. Axial FSE T2-weighted images at the level of the lower third vagina (*C*), middle third vagina (*D*), and upper third vagina (*E*) are obtained at rest. Although the lowest level (*C*) may appear to have normal relations between the lateral vagina and the pelvic side wall (*arrows*), it becomes apparent that this relation is distracted at higher levels, and the vagina is folded in on itself and no longer closely apposed to the pelvic side walls (*D, E; arrows*). (*F*) Normally, the vaginal cuff, representing the resection margins in the patient after hysterectomy, should also remain apposed to the pelvic side walls laterally, and the mesorectal fascia posteriorly (*F, black arrows*), with the ureters passing anteriorly (*F, white arrows*), but the vagina is drawn medially and inferiorly in this patient. Also note that the levator ani (*C, D; arrows*) appears intact although the patient has severe prolapse. Cx, cervix; R, rectum.

their patients with POP and incontinence before and after surgical treatments.

Abdominal and vaginal approaches

Traditionally, approaches to surgical repair of pelvic floor defects and prolapse have been approached by way of a transabdominal or transvaginal approach. Until the late 1980s, the most common procedures used for correcting multiple defects were vaginal hysterectomy, bilateral sacrospinous ligament vault suspension, vaginal paravaginal repair, and needle urethropexy or an autologous sling [15]. If the abdominal route was chosen, abdominal hysterectomy, Burch urethropexy, or an autologous sling was used. The surgical approach largely depended on the surgeon responsible and the identified pelvic support defects. With the abdominal approach, the chance for successful surgical outcome is twice as

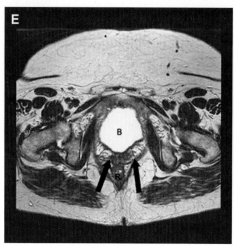
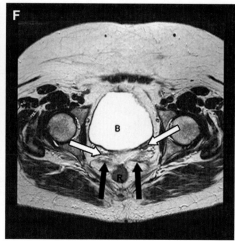

Fig. 2 (continued)

great and there are benefits in complex individuals, those with short vaginas, or those desiring future pregnancy.

From the perspective of MR imaging

The authors propose that combining a surgical understanding of the pelvic support structures and repair strategies with the soft tissue analysis obtained by optimized MR imaging may facilitate an improved documentation and understanding of the surgical mechanisms of treatment. The following describes a methodologic approach with clinical examples.

MR imaging technique

The patient is asked to void only partially before the study, because although overdistention of the bladder may prevent uterine and small bowel descent, a partially distended bladder improves visualization of prolapse of the bladder and vagina. Imaging is then performed with a combination of T2-weighted single-shot fast spin echo (SST2; for speed and resistance to motion-related deterioration), T2-weighted fast spin echo (FSE; for maximized soft tissue detail), and T1-weighted gradient-recalled echo (GRE; particularly in postoperative cases to evaluate for complications like infection or scarring). Dynamic images with the patient at rest and straining may be acquired using SST2. Sagittal and axial images are essential for a complete evaluation. Surface coils are also essential and maximize the signal-to-noise ratio for optimized soft tissue delineation. Internal coils have not been favored because of a combination of patient discomfort, mechanical tissue distortion, and insufficient field of view.

Adequate comprehensive evaluation of the pelvic soft tissues can be obtained using the SST2

technique [16,17]. Typical imaging parameters include a partial Fourier processing of k-space to achieve shorter acquisition time. This method is performed in two dimensions to achieve slice-by-slice acquisition that is relatively rapid and insensitive to motion-related deterioration. The repetition time (TR) is set to around 1000 to 1200 milliseconds but is effectively increased by using interleaving to reduce cross-talk effects that may diminish the signal-to-noise ratio. The echo time (TE) is adjusted to 80 to 100 milliseconds to achieve optimal T2-weighted contrast. Surface phased-array coils are implemented to optimize signal but also to allow use of parallel processing. Although parallel processing does not affect the overall acquisition time for SST2, it significantly improves image quality by compacting the echo spacing. SST2 can be acquired in at least the axial and sagittal planes, but the authors also acquire it in the coronal plane to ensure comprehensive visualization of the potentially important soft tissue disruptions associated with pelvic floor instability and incontinence. Fat suppression is generally not useful for this analysis, because the high-signal fat acts to provide contrast against the low signal from bones, muscles, gynecologic soft tissues, and ligaments.

In addition to SST2, the authors acquire a standard FSE image at relatively higher resolution over the lower pelvis. This technique requires approximately 4 minutes to acquire images at near 400 to 500 phase lines of resolution, typically with a 4-mm slice thickness. FSE images are sensitive to motion-related image degradation, and thus tend to be useful only in the lower pelvis, where breathing-related motion is minimal. The authors have found this sequence helpful to delineate the relation between the lateral wall of the vagina and the pelvic side walls.

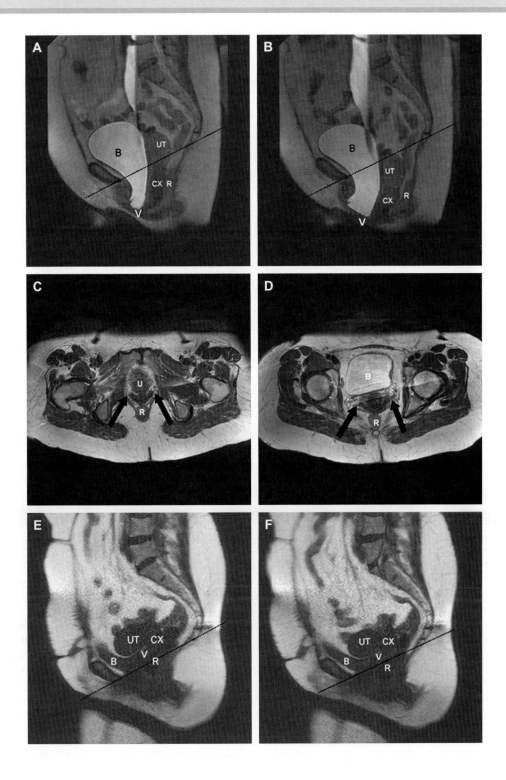

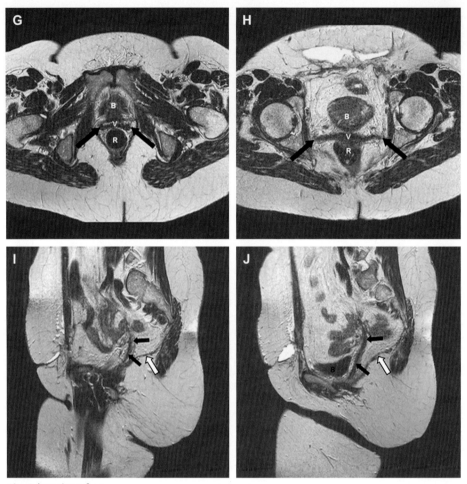

Fig. 3 (continued)

Contrast-enhanced three-dimensional (3D) GRE may be useful for further evaluation and localization of gynecologic structures, particularly the vagina. The authors have not found these images to be necessary or helpful for delineation of the gynecologic soft tissues in the setting of pelvic floor instability, however. The ligamentous soft tissues also are rendered inconspicuous using this technique. Other uses include evaluation of complications, such as may arise in the postsurgical patient, for assessment of inflammation, infection, or abscess formation or for evaluation of fibrotic changes.

The authors have found that higher field 3-T systems may yield similarly high-quality SST2 sequences. The increased signal achievable on 3 T is particularly beneficial when implementing the

Fig. 3. Multiparous patient with the uterus intact but with bilateral uterosacral ligament disruption and prolapse before (*A–D*) and after (*E, F*) bilateral repair. Presurgical images show marked prolapse below the pubo-coccygeal line (*A, B; dotted arrow*) of the rectum (R) and vagina (V) at rest (*A*) and stress (*B*). Note that the cervix (Cx) is situated low and anterior in regard to the sacrum. (*C, D*) Axial images show that the vagina is pulled away from the pelvic side walls and folded. This is less evident on the axial image through the lower third of the vagina (*C, arrows*) and more evident on the higher axial slice through the middle third vagina (*D, arrows*). After bilateral uterosacral ligament repair, there is diminished prolapse below the pubo-coccygeal line (*E, F; dotted line*) and approximation of the lateral vaginal walls to the pelvic side walls with tightening of the vagina (*G, H; arrows*). Sagittal images slicing through the pelvic side walls on the left (*I, black arrows*) and right (*J, black arrows*) sides show the surgically thickened bands of the reconstituted uterosacral ligaments. The levator ani is indicated (*I, J; white arrow*) for reference, and has a more normal horizontal position compared to the presurgical images (compare to *A, B*). B, bladder; UT, urethra.

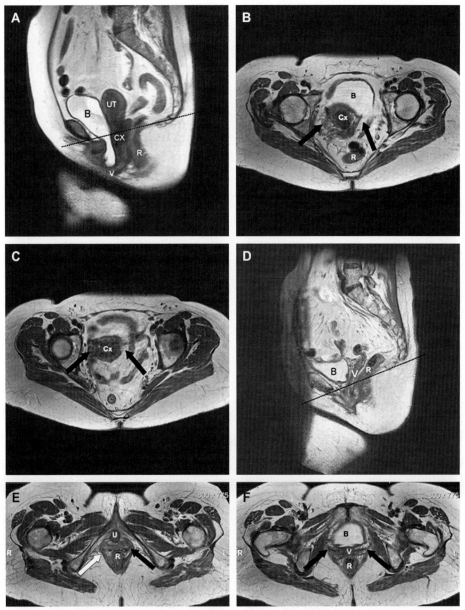

Fig. 4. Multiparous patient with severe prolapse attributable to unilateral uterosacral ligament injury before (*A–C*) and after (*D–F*). (*A*) Sagittal SST2 image shows severe prolapse below the pubo-coccygeal line (*A, dotted line*) of the bladder (B), vagina (V), and rectum (R). The vagina is being pulled down underneath the bladder, and the vagina and urethra (UT) are folding while curving anteriorly and superiorly, maintaining connection with the undersurface of the symphysis pubis. (*B, C*) The axial T2-weighted images show that the cervix (Cx) is pulled to the right side of the pelvis with relative preservation of the right uterosacral ligament (USL) and disruption of the left USL (*black arrows*). After hysterectomy and unilateral left USL repair (*D–F*), the sagittal SST2 image shows marked improvement in prolapse below the pubo-coccygeal line (*D, dotted line*), with pulling up and straightening of the vagina (*E, F*). The lateral walls of the vagina are well apposed to the lateral pelvic walls (*E, F; black arrows*) and to the levator ani (*E, white arrow*).

standard FSE T2-weighted technique, however. For a similar acquisition time and similar parameters, the additional signal can be converted to nearly a doubling of the in-plane resolution with a similar signal-to-noise ratio in the final image. The authors typically acquire images with 800 phase lines of resolution on the 3-T system.

To achieve an understanding of the dynamic process of pelvic floor instability, the authors routinely acquire sagittal SST2 sequences as a midsagittal series of images. These images are acquired in only one slice position and are repeated while the patient is instructed to perform repeated Valsalva maneuvers. This achieves an elevation of the intra-abdominal pressure and exacerbates findings related to prolapse of the gynecologic soft tissues, rectum, and bladder. The resistance of SST2 to motion deterioration results in a series of time-resolved images that show motion between each of the images, which is best displayed as a cinematic loop. The image quality of each image is well maintained individually, however.

Image analysis of normal subjects

Viewed in conjunction with directly observed surgical anatomy, the region of the uterosacral ligament may be depicted in the normal subject (see Fig. 1), which is shown as connective tissue extending around the cervix and lateral vaginal fornices and outwardly toward and along the pelvic side walls. This is best visualized on axial and coronal images and represents the components of level I support. The middle and lower axial vaginal images (see Fig. 1B, C) show the relation between the lateral vaginal wall and the pelvic side wall, representing the region forming level II support. The anterior vagina along the posteroinferior wall of the bladder, as shown in Fig. 1G, represents the location of the pubocervical fascia. The posterior vaginal wall, as also shown in Fig. 1G, demarcates the course of the rectovaginal fascia. Although the soft tissue margins between the bladder, vagina, and rectum are well demonstrated, the specific visualization of the connective tissue comprising these fascias is not seen as separate structures.

Image analysis of abnormal symptomatic subjects

In symptomatic patients, the authors have found good correlation between surgically determined disruption of the uterosacral ligaments and the MR imaging findings (Figs. 2–4). These new principles correlating MR imaging with surgical and physical examination findings are discussed using the following case presentations.

Case presentations

Case 1

This patient is multiparous, had a prior hysterectomy, and was found to have marked pelvic prolapse and bilateral disruption of the uterosacral ligaments (see Fig. 2). The images show the contribution of the rest-stress SST2 images, with the magnitude of prolapse being significantly greater after the patient is asked to perform a Valsalva maneuver. A partially filled bladder facilitates this visualization. In addition, the SST2 images retain good quality, even

though the patient's abdomen is in motion during the acquisition. The separation of the vaginal lateral margins and infolding away from the pelvic side walls is in keeping with disruption of the pelvic lateral attachments, including the level I and II support structures. A hysterectomy may have contributed to loss of the integrity of level I support structures.

Case 2

This patient has a presentation similar to case 1, but the uterus remains intact (see Fig. 3). There is evidence of cystocele and rectocele on sagittal imaging and apical prolapse with descent of the vaginal apex. As for the previous patient, bilateral repair of the uterosacral ligaments significantly reconstituted the vaginal and cervical positions within the pelvis and mechanically supports the urethra and bladder and corrects the cystocele. As in the prior case, although only partial reconstitution of the rectum is noted, the patient's symptoms were corrected. These findings help to demonstrate that it is not essential to repair the uterus but that the reconstituted support of the vagina and cervix, level I support structures, may alone represent the essential mechanical support necessary to correct the urinary symptoms. Rectal symptoms seem to require at least partial repositioning of the rectum and reformation of the rectal angulation that normally is seen between the proximal rectum and the distal rectum and anus.

Case 3

Fig. 4 shows the results of asymmetric unilateral disruption of the uterosacral ligament, the level I support structure, on the left side only. The remaining intact right uterosacral ligament is responsible for pulling the cervix over to the unopposed right side. These findings help to demonstrate the significance of the uterosacral ligament for supporting the cervix and vagina normally. Recognizing this disruption helps to guide the surgical repair approach so as to concentrate on correcting the disrupted left side. The presence of a large cystocele and rectocele represents imaging evidence for disruption of level II and III support. The use of MR imaging in this case is to document further the mechanical relations of the pelvic soft tissues and to demonstrate technical success of surgery.

Summary

Pelvic MR imaging using the combination of motion-insensitive SST2 and high soft tissue resolution standard T2-weighted FSE techniques has helped to identify soft tissue abnormalities that directly correlate with the clinical and intraoperative findings related to pelvic floor prolapse. In particular, the authors have shown that pelvic MR imaging has the ability to identify changes related to uterosacral ligament disruption and to document the corrective changes after surgical repair of this ligament. In the future, pelvic MR imaging is expected to play a progressively larger role in preoperative planning for complex or uncertain cases and for more detailed evaluation of repair in cases that do not show good symptomatic response. Pelvic MR imaging should also help to document and advance knowledge of surgical repair methodology. Education may be affected significantly by pelvic MR imaging in a field that has become defined by numerous surgical repair techniques between different centers but with few objective methods for documentation of outcomes.

References

[1] Palmer MH, Fitzgerald S. Urinary incontinence in working women: a comparison study. J Womens Health (Larchmt) 2002;11:879–88.

[2] Rovner ES, Ginsberg DA, Raz S. Female stress urinary incontinence clinical guidelines panel summary report on surgical management of female stress urinary incontinence [letter to the editor]. J Urol 1998;159:1646–7.

[3] Richardson AC, Edmonds PB, Williams NL. Treatment of stress urinary incontinence due to paravaginal fascial defect. Obstet Gynecol 1981;57:357–62.

[4] Miller KL. Stress urinary incontinence in women: review and update on neurological control. J Womens Health (Larchmt) 2005;14:595–608.

[5] Schneider G, Uder M. Contrast-enhanced magnetic resonance body imaging 5. Top Magn Reson Imaging 2003;14:403–25.

[6] Morakkabati-Spitz N, Gieseke J, Kuhl C, et al. 3.0-T high-field magnetic resonance imaging of the female pelvis: preliminary experiences. Eur Radiol 2005;15:639–44.

[7] Handa VL, Pannu HK, Siddique S, et al. Architectural differences in the bony pelvis of women with and without pelvic floor disorders. Obstet Gynecol 2003;102:1283–90.

[8] Tunn R, Delancey JOl, Howard D, et al. Anatomic variations in the levator ani muscle, endopelvic fascia, and urethra in nulliparas evaluated by magnetic resonance imaging. Am J Obstet Gynecol 2003;188:116–21.

[9] Maubon A, Aubard Y, Berkane V, et al. Magnetic resonance imaging of the pelvic floor. Abdom Imaging 2003;28:217–25.

[10] Stoker J, Rociu E, Bosch JLHR, et al. High-resolution endovaginal MR imaging in stress urinary incontinence. Eur Radiol 2003;13: 2031–7.

[11] Chou Q, DeLancey JOL. A structured system to evaluate urethral support anatomy in magnetic resonance imaging. Am J Obstet Gynecol 2001; 185:44–50.

[12] Deval B, Vulierme MP, Poilpot S, et al. [Imaging pelvic floor prolapse]. J Gynecol Obstet Biol Reprod 2003;32:22–9.

[13] Singh K, Jakab M, Reid WMN, et al. Three-dimensional magnetic resonance imaging assessment of levator ani morphologic features in different grades of prolapse. Am J Obstet Gynecol 2003;188:910–5.

[14] Marshall VF, Marchetti AA, Kranz KE. The correction of stress incontinence by simple vesicourethral suspension. Surg Gynecol Obstet 1949;88: 509–18.

[15] Stanton SL. Female pelvic reconstructive surgery. Springer; 2003.

[16] Tunn R, DeLancey JO, Quint EE. Visibility of pelvic organ support system structures in magnetic resonance images without an endovaginal coil. Am J Obstet Gynecol 2001;184: 1156–63.

[17] Martin DR, Friel HT, Danrad R, et al. Approach to abdominal imaging at 1.5 Tesla and optimization at 3 Tesla. Magn Reson Imaging Clin N Am 2005;13:241–54.

ELSEVIER
SAUNDERS

MAGNETIC
RESONANCE
IMAGING CLINICS

Magn Reson Imaging Clin N Am 14 (2007) 537–544

MR Imaging of the Female Pelvis at 3T

Shahid M. Hussain, MD, PhD[a],*, Indra C. van den Bos, MD[b],
Jennifer M. Oliveto, MD[a], Diego R. Martin, MD, PhD[c]

- Parallel MR imaging and its importance for pelvic imaging at 3.0T
- Female pelvic MR imaging at 3.0T: general considerations
  Signal-to-noise ratio
  Radio frequency power deposition
  Chemical shift and susceptibility artifact

  Radio frequency coils
  Other issues, such as dielectric resonances, B1 field inhomogeneities, and the shape of the anatomy at 3.0T
- Female pelvic MR imaging at 3.0T
- Summary
- References

The recent development and approval of the transmit-receive body coil and dedicated torso phased-array radio frequency (RF) receive coil for 3.0 Tesla (T) MR imaging systems have promoted a move toward higher-field body MR imaging, including pelvic MR imaging. The female pelvis in particular is an anatomic area that may benefit from the advantages of high-field systems. With about double the signal-to-noise ratio (SNR) of a 1.5T system, 3.0T MR systems can improve image quality and image acquisition speed substantially. Potentially, 3.0T can deliver a $\sqrt{2}$ improvement in resolution in the same acquisition time as a comparable study at 1.5T; a half-slice thickness with identical coverage; or a fourfold speed-up in scanning time for identical resolution settings [1].

For the clinical application and further development of body MR imaging at 3.0T, a number of other important developments include (1) improved coil design with multiple overlapping coil elements

(eg, 16–32 elements), which provide a higher SNR in combination with sufficient depth; (2) a greater number of coils in combination with a higher B0 (main magnetic field), which allows the application of higher acceleration factors for parallel imaging for higher spatial and temporal resolution in the pelvis; (3) improved bandwidth per receiver channel (3 MHz), with advances in digital electronics for faster readouts and faster reconstructions of k-space data sets; (4) increased gradient performance (from gradients of <10 mT/m with switching rates of >1 ms, to gradients of >50 mT/m with switching rates in the order of 100 μs), which can achieve lower repetition time (TR) and echo time (TE) values and allow better spatial and temporal coverage, and can reduce drastically the dead time periods during which no MR signal is acquired [1].

Several vendors suggest that anatomy that is difficult to image at lower field strengths, such as the female and male pelvis, may be imaged without

[a] Department of Radiology, University of Nebraska Medical Center, 981045 Nebraska Medical Center, Omaha, NE 68198-1045, USA
[b] Department of Radiology, Erasmus Medical Center, Dr Molewaterplein 40, 3015 GD Rotterdam, The Netherlands
[c] Department of Radiology, Emory University School of Medicine, Emory University Hospital, 1365 Clifton Road NE, Atlanta, GA 30322, USA
* Corresponding author.
E-mail address: smhussain@unmc.edu (S.M. Hussain).

1064-9689/07/$ – see front matter © 2007 Elsevier Inc. All rights reserved.
mri.theclinics.com

doi:10.1016/j.mric.2007.01.008

additional intraluminal coils, significantly reducing patient discomfort and preparation time.

Specific absorption rate (SAR) management is an important issue for body MR imaging at 3.0T [1]. Increased SAR deposition reduces the number of slices per TR and, potentially, can lengthen the examination times at 3.0T. Because breath holding is not an important issue in the pelvis, it may not affect the examination times as much as in the upper abdomen. However, other items, such as B1 (local magnetic field) inhomogeneities and dielectric resonances, may cause suboptimal fat suppression and other artifacts, especially in the pelvis.

A number of excellent papers have already been published that provide a superb description and illustration of MR imaging of the female pelvis anatomy and various disease entities at 1.5T [2–5]. In this article, the authors present their initial experience with optimization of sequences for MR imaging of the female pelvis at 3.0T and include a short description of parallel imaging because of its importance for imaging at 3.0T. They also provide some general remarks comparing some of the physical properties of 3.0T, discuss some of the challenges during sequence optimization for the female pelvis at 3.0T, and give examples of female pelvic abnormalities.

Parallel MR imaging and its importance for pelvic imaging at 3.0T

The key feature of parallel MR (pMR) imaging methods is the application of multiple independent receiver coils with distinct sensitivities across the object being imaged [6–9]. In conventional MR imaging, the role of phased-array coils was merely to improve the SNR, whereas in pMR imaging, the phased-array coils are used either to reduce the scan time or to improve the spatial resolution. Other important applications of parallel imaging include (1) reduced effective inter-echo spacing (less image blurring and image distortion in echo-train, spin-echo, and echo-planar imaging [EPI] [eg, high-quality, single-shot EPI of the pelvis]), and (2) reduced SAR due to shorter echo-trains, which is important for the optimization of pelvic MR imaging sequences at 3.0T.

Female pelvic MR imaging at 3.0T: general considerations

Image quality, reproducibility of image quality, and good conspicuity of disease require the use of sequences that are robust and reliable and that avoid artifacts [1–5]. Maximizing these principles to achieve high-quality diagnostic pelvic MR images usually requires the use of fast scanning techniques, with the overall intention of generating images with consistent image quality that demonstrate consistent display of disease processes. Another advantage of using fast scanning techniques is that, when beneficial to diagnostic yield, a greater number of individual sequences can be employed within a reasonably short total examination time. This approach contributes to one of the major strengths of MR imaging, which is comprehensive information on disease processes.

The main goals of female pelvic MR imaging include (1) multi-planar display of the zonal pelvic anatomy, mainly with high resolution T2-weighted images, (2) detection and characterization of diffuse and focal lesions, (3) detection and characterization of congenital female pelvic anomalies, and (4) follow-up of disease processes. Currently, in many institutions, female pelvic MR imaging is used mainly as a problem-solving modality and combines the high intrinsic, soft-tissue contrast with high spatial resolution to display disease. Gadolinium-enhanced dynamic imaging is applied to patients who have suspect or known neoplasms of the female pelvis [2–5].

A major advantage of a 3.0T system compared with a 1.5T system is that the SNR at 3.0T is about two times higher. Currently, state-of-the-art 3.0T MR imaging systems can be equipped with eight-element torso phased-array coils and parallel MR imaging capability. The availability of pMR imaging at 3.0T is essential for reducing SAR. Potentially, eight-element torso phased-array coils facilitate larger field of view (FOV) and larger anatomic coverage, in combination with better SNR distribution over the region of interest, compared with four-channel, phased-array torso coils at 1.5T and 3.0T; this advantage may be particularly important for staging the female pelvic malignancies. Before the goal of female pelvic MR imaging at 3.0T can be achieved, several issues must be considered.

Signal-to-noise ratio

At 3.0T, SNR is improved by a factor of two, compared with 1.5T [6–9]. In clinical settings, further development of the coil technology will be important to take full advantage of the higher SNR for female pelvic MR imaging.

Radio frequency power deposition

To excite the protons at 3.0T, RF pulses with four times higher energy (higher B1) are needed. Increased B1 energy results in more RF heating and higher SAR [6–9]. According to Food and Drug Administration guidelines, the SAR thresholds are 2 W/kg in normal mode and 4 W/kg body weight in the first-level controlled mode [10–16]. The limitation of SAR is greatest for RF-intensive sequences, including all sequences based on fast spin-echo (FSE) readouts. At 3.0T, these limitations result in a fewer number of slices per TR (smaller anatomic coverage).

A number of solutions can be considered, including parallel imaging, specialized RF pulses, RF pulses with reduced flip angle, hyper-echo mechanism, and "transition between pseudo steady states" (TRAPS) [17–20]. FSE scans are usually RF-intensive. Generally, to reduce SAR, the refocusing angles of the FSE train (180°) are lowered (110°–160°) to make it possible to scan an adequate number of slices. Nonetheless, lowering the refocusing angles has a penalty on SNR. Hennig and Scheffler [17] have devised a new spin-refocusing strategy that maintains the benefits of FSE by employing echoes of echoes (hence the name, hyper-echoes), preserving SNR as in conventional FSE sequences but with dramatically reduced SAR values (reductions up to 70%–90%).

The principle behind hyper-echoes is not straightforward. In essence, a sequence of refocusing RF pulses, played with arbitrary flip angles, phase, and gradient pulses, following an initial 90° RF excitation pulse, will refocus to a full echo after the application of a 180° inversion pulse, if the initial sequence of RF refocusing pulses is applied in reverse order with negated amplitudes and phases and the same gradient pulsing scheme. The signal intensity of the generated hyper-echo can be thought of as the addition of all individual coherence pathways generated by each RF pulse (mixing of transverse and longitudinal magnetization components and generation of stimulated echoes) at the time of the hyper-echo. In general, relaxation and diffusion effects accumulate between RF pulses, and these provide additional modulation of the amplitude of the hyper-echo. Usually, to obtain T2 contrast similar to that obtained with FSE, the effective TE is increased. Frank and colleagues [19] have taken advantage of the increased SNR of hyper-echoes to produce a sequence with greater diffusion contrast. The TRAPS approach is based on the observation that the static pseudo steady state (PSS) for a given refocusing flip angle, which yields the maximum attainable signal, is extremely robust against flip angle variations. TRAPS offers a very simple way to reduce RF power deposition significantly for FSE imaging. By using high flip angles only for the important data encoding for the central part of k-space, a considerable reduction in RF power is achieved. The essential step for retrieving the full signal is the preparation of the static PSS. Both hyper-echo and TRAPS may be used to reduce SAR without any appreciable loss in image quality for various applications [17,18]. Recently, the

authors showed the application of variable-rate-selective excitation (VERSE)-RF pulses for increased slice coverage in fat-suppressed T2-weighted fast-spin-echo imaging at 3.0T. They showed that the use of VERSE-RF pulses provides a 38% to 58% increase in slice coverage with homogenous fat suppression and good overall image quality (Van den Bosen, unpublished data, 2007). They also evaluated diffusion-weighted, black-blood EPI (BBEPI) as a potential alternative to SAR-intensive, echo-train, spin-echo sequences at 3.0T. The optimized BBEPI provided T2-weighted images with good overall image quality, homogenous fat suppression, and high SNR (unpublished data). Geometric distortions in BBEPI were acceptable.

Chemical shift and susceptibility artifact

Higher chemical shifts and susceptibility may result in artifacts on every sequence [6]. Chemical shift artifacts can be reduced by using higher readout bandwidths, and susceptibility effects can be decreased by shorter TE values. Scaling bandwidth in excitation will affect SAR and influencing readout bandwidth in acquisition (readout) will change SNR. Higher chemical shift, however, is advantageous for MR spectroscopy (fourfold faster and twofold better spectral separation for the same voxel size as 1.5T), which may have an application in the characterization of female pelvic masses.

Radio frequency coils

At 3.0T, fewer coils are available, in comparison with 1.5T. Phased-array coils with an increased number of coil elements have several advantages, including (1) larger anatomic coverage with sufficient SNR over the entire field-of-view; (2) more coil elements, allowing higher parallel imaging acceleration factors; (3) higher acceleration factors, allowing faster imaging with high matrices, and reduced echo-spacing for less blurring and image distortion. Currently, the eight-element torso phased-array coil allows larger FOV, and higher pMR imaging acceleration factors of up to three. Larger anatomic coverage is beneficial for combined abdominopelvic imaging (eg, for the staging of female pelvic malignancies).

Other issues, such as dielectric resonances, B1 field inhomogeneities, and the shape of the anatomy at 3.0T

The RF wavelength is reduced at 3.0T because of the higher operational frequency of 128 MHz (compared with 64 MHz at 1.5T). In tissues, the effective wavelength is reduced further by permittivity because this decreases with increasing frequency. The effective wavelength for the pelvis at 3.0T is reduced to about 30 cm, such that the object is in the order

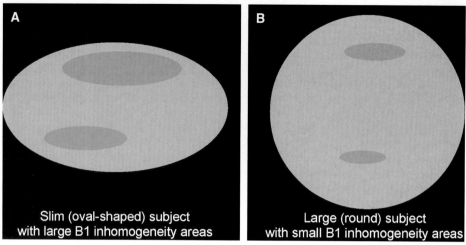

Fig. 1. Signal loss due to the B1 field inhomogeneities based on the shape and size of the female pelvis. The slim (oval-shaped) subject (*A*) will show more signal loss than a large (round) subject (*B*).

of the wavelength. In addition, the conductivity increases with frequency, and generates eddy currents that act against the applied external RF pulses, resulting in B1-inhomogeneity [21–23]. B1 inhomogeneities, which cause variations in the signal distribution over the region of interest, appear to be related to the shape and size of the anatomy (Figs. 1 and 2). For instance, at the level of the pelvis, B1 inhomogeneities cause darkening in the anterior and posterior parts of the abdomen and pelvis. The B1 inhomogeneities, in combination with the nature of the fat suppression and the refocusing pulses in echo-train, spin-echo sequences (Shinnar-Le Roux pulses), may also be responsible for the poor quality of fat suppression. To reduce SAR and acquire T2-weighted sequences with better fat suppression, alternative fat suppression techniques and T2-weighted imaging sequences have to be optimized at 3.0T, such as EPI with spectral-spatial water excitation pulse. The authors have

extensive experience with a T2-weighted, diffusion-weighted BBEPI sequence [24] and their initial experience suggests that BBEPI works at 3.0T as well, with good fat suppression (Fig. 3). Better fat suppression with BBEPI is facilitated mainly by the lack of refocusing pulses. Other measures include the use of adiabatic pulses with B1-insensitive RF pulses (disadvantage: such pulses last longer and cause more power deposition) and phase cycling (disadvantage: scan time is increased) [21].

Female pelvic MR imaging at 3.0T

Female pelvic MR imaging at 3.0T should facilitate at least the sequences performed at 1.5T at the authors' institutions [2–5]. The state-of-the-art female pelvic MR imaging protocol at 1.5T includes a set of sequences: (1) axial, sagittal, and coronal single-shot fast spin-echo (SSFSE) for planning other sequences and for overview of the anatomy; (2)

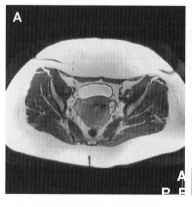

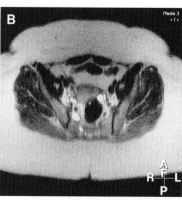

Fig. 2. Axial T2-weighted FSE images at 3.0T in a slim (*A*) and an obese (*B*) volunteer demonstrate the signal loss due to the B1 field inhomogeneities.

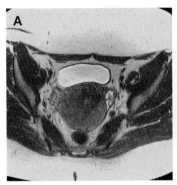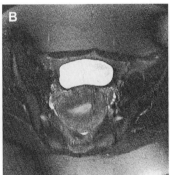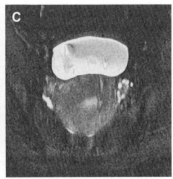

Fig. 3. Axial T2-weighted FSE image without fat suppression (*A*), with suboptimal fat suppression due to B1 field inhomogeneities and other effects (*B*), and diffusion-weighted T2-weighted EPI with complete homogeneous fat suppression and good overall image quality with minimal image distortion at 3.0T (*C*).

high-resolution axial FSE, with and without fat suppression, for more detailed zonal anatomy of the uterus, cervix, vagina, and ovaries; (3) high-resolution sagittal or oblique-sagittal (long axis of the uterus) to evaluate the zonal anatomy of the uterus and to detect and characterize uterine abnormalities, including anomalies; and (4) dynamic, gadolinium-enhanced (precontrast, arterial phase, venous phase, delayed phase), three-dimensional (3D) gradient-echo sequences for further detection and characterization of female pelvic malignancies. Occasionally, the authors employ chemical shift sequences to detect small amounts of fat, for instance in ovarian lesions.

At 3.0T, a similar approach should be adopted with the use of the higher SNR to improve the image quality. The authors' initial experience demonstrates that high-quality female pelvic MR imaging can be performed in patients who have a wide range of abnormalities (Fig. 4). Typically, the SSFSE sequences can take advantage of the higher SNR, in combination with parallel imaging. Parallel

imaging reduces the inter-echo spacing and hence, results in less blurring in the images. High-resolution FSE sequences can be obtained with higher matrices for improved in-plane resolution. At 3.0T, however, both SSFSE and FSE sequences are SAR-intensive and result in a smaller number of slices per TR, compared with 1.5T using similar sequence parameters. The authors' initial experience shows that a wide range of female pelvic abnormalities can be imaged at 3.0T (Figs. 5–7).

Currently, the greatest advantage of the higher SNR of 3.0T, eight-channel torso phased-array coils, and the possibility of higher (>2) pMR imaging acceleration factors is applicable to 3D gradient echo gadolinium-enhanced sequences. Typically, a 3D gradient echo sequence is performed with minimum TR and TE and a flip angle between 10° and 15°. The flip angle is related to the TR. With a minimum TR, the flip angle can also be relatively low. Because the TR and TE of these sequences have minimum values, the flip angle mainly determines the contrast in the images. With 3D, a volume, instead

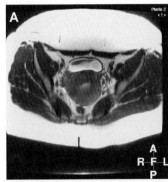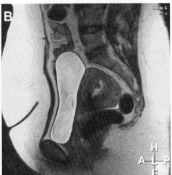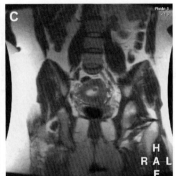

Fig. 4. Axial (*A*), sagittal (*B*), and coronal (*C*) T2-weighted FSE images at 3.0T with good overview and detail of the female pelvic anatomy in a relatively large subject.

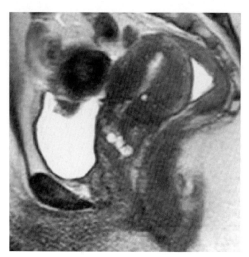

Fig. 5. Sagittal T2-weighted FSE image at 3.0T shows nabothian cysts at the level of the cervix and diffuse adenomyosis with thickened junctional zone containing punctate high signal.

of individual slices, is acquired. Subsequently, the volume is divided into thin sections. Several advantages of 3D versus 2D gradient echo sequences are

1. Higher inherent SNR than the 2D gradient echo sequences
2. Higher in-plane resolution with larger matrices (>320 × >380);
3. Thinner sections (2–5 mm) for higher through-plane resolution with the possibility of reformats in other planes; thin sections are often possible because of interpolation of the MR data in the z-direction;
4. Homogenous fat suppression (most vendors apply segmented fat suppression [ie, fat suppression pulse is applied after every *nth* k-space

line (n can typically be up to 60–70)]), which allows scan times that are still short enough to perform breath-hold imaging with fat suppression; this is not possible with 2D gradient echo sequences because of the increase in scan time (>30 seconds) if a fat suppression pulse is applied for a similar anatomic coverage;

The enhancement of vessels and tissues with gadolinium is more obvious because of the fat-suppressed nature of the sequence and the increased sensitivity of tissues to gadolinium at 3.0T [25].

Summary

This article illustrates that female pelvic MR imaging is feasible at 3.0T, but needs further optimization. The image quality seems to be good for several important sequences, including SSFSE, EPI, and gadolinium-enhanced, 3D, T1-weighted sequences. The authors' initial experience with abdominal MR imaging at 3.0T also shows that several technical problems have to be solved.

Despite the inherent increased SNR at 3.0T (theoretically on the order of two with respect to 1.5T), increased tissue T1 relaxation times, quality of fat suppression, higher SAR, chemical shift, dielectric resonances, and B1 inhomogeneity, larger susceptibility and geometric distortions must be considered. Therefore, relevant sequences must be evaluated and optimized to obtain the highest yield with all the difficulties mentioned. In this respect, the recent implementation of specialized, shaped RF pulses, such as VERSE, have reduced SAR figures and, hence, increased slice efficiency per unit time. Also, the increased SNR at 3.0T can be used to relieve some imaging restrictions through the use of parallel imaging and partial Fourier, and yet provide good image quality and volume coverage

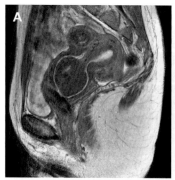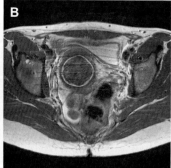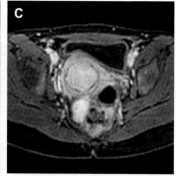

Fig. 6. Axial (*A*) and sagittal (*B*) T2-weighted FSE images at 3.0T show a large pedunculated fibroid with predominantly low signal intensity. Axial fat-suppressed, gadolinium-enhanced, 3D, T1-weighted gradient-echo image at 3.0T (*C*) shows persistent enhancement, confirming the benign nature of the lesion.

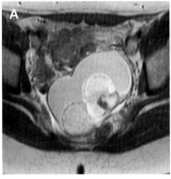 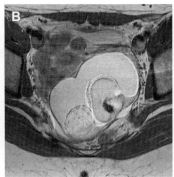 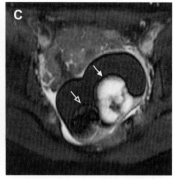

Fig. 7. Axial SSFSE (*A*) and high-resolution FSE (*B*) images at 3.0T show a large complex fluid-filled cystic lesion with solid components. Axial fat-suppressed, gadolinium-enhanced, 3D, T1-weighted gradient-echo image at 3.0T (*C*) shows enhancement of the solid component (*solid arrow*). A part of the lesion contains fat and shows signal loss caused by the fat suppression (*open arrow*). The findings are consistent with an ovarian cystic teratoma.

with multiple imaging sequences, including diffusion-weighted BBEPI protocols [26–28].

Future technical improvement and sequence optimization at 3.0T should focus on (1) further improvement of RF receive coils with an increased number of coil elements and channels; (2) application of parallel imaging with larger acceleration factors; (3) SAR management; (4) fat suppression issues; and (5) chemical shift imaging. With these technical developments and implementation, new applications will emerge that will improve the diagnostic capability of abdominal MR imaging at 1.5T and 3.0T, including female pelvic MR imaging.

References

[1] Hussain SM, Wielopolski PA, Martin DR. Abdominal magnetic resonance imaging at 3.0T: problem or a promise for the future? Top Magn Reson Imaging 2005;16:325–35.

[2] Outwater EK, Dunton CJ. Imaging of the ovary and adnexa: clinical issues and applications of MR imaging. Radiology 1995;194:1–18.

[3] Outwater EK, Mitchell DG. Magnetic resonance imaging techniques in the pelvis. Magn Reson Imaging Clin N Am 1994;2:161–88.

[4] Audet P, Pressacco J, Burken M, et al. MR imaging of female pelvic malignancies. Magn Reson Imaging Clin N Am 2000;8:887–914.

[5] Brown MA, Sirlin CB. Female pelvis. Magn Reson Imaging Clin N Am 2005;13:381–95.

[6] Campeau NG, Huston J, Bernstein MA, et al. Magnetic resonance angiography at 3.0 Tesla: initial clinical experience. Top Magn Reson Imaging 2001;12:183–204.

[7] Norris DG. High field human imaging. J Magn Reson Imaging 2003;18:519–29.

[8] Watkins RD, Schenk JF, Rohling KW, et al. Whole body RF coil for 3 tesla MRI systems. Proceeding of the International Society of Magnetic Resonance in Medicine 2001;9:1123.

[9] Roberts S, Freeman A, Murphy P, et al. High definition whole body imaging at 3tesla. Proceeding of the International Society of Magnetic Resonance in Medicine 2001;9:2013.

[10] Martin DR, Friel HT, Danrad R, et al. Approach to abdominal imaging at 1.5 tesla and optimization at 3 tesla. Magn Reson Imaging Clin N Am 2005;13:241–54.

[11] Takahashi M, Uematsu H, Hatabu H. MR imaging at high magnetic fields. Eur J Radiol 2003; 46:45–52.

[12] Sodickson DK, Manning WJ. Simultaneous acquisition of spatial harmonics (SMASH): fast imaging with radio-frequency coil arrays. Magn Reson Med 1997;38:591–603.

[13] Pruessmann KP, Weiger M, Scheidigger MB, et al. SENSE: sensitivity encoding for fast MRI. Magn Reson Med 1999;42:952–62.

[14] Griswold MA, Jakob PM, Heidemann RM, et al. Generalized auto-calibrating partially parallel acquisition (GRAPPA). Magn Reson Med 2002; 47:1202–10.

[15] Hutchinson M, Raff U. Fast MRI data acquisition using multiple detectors. Magn Reson Med 1988; 6:87–91.

[16] Brix B, Seebass M, Hellwig G, et al. Estimation of heat transfer and temperature rise in partial-body regions during MR procedures: an analytical approach with respect to safety considerations. Magn Reson Imaging 2002;20:65–76.

[17] Hennig J, Scheffler K. Hyperechoes. Magn Reson Med 2001;46:6–12.

[18] Hennig J, Weigel M, Scheffler K. Multiecho sequences with variable refocusing flip angles: optimization of signal behavior using smooth transition between pseudo steady states (TRAPS). Magn Reson Med 2003;49:527–35.

[19] Frank LR, Wong EC, Liu TT, et al. Increased diffusion sensitivity with hyperechoes. Magn Reson Med 2003;49:1096–105.

[20] Busse RF, Zur Y, Body XL. Lower SAR yields improved coverage with VERSE and modulated angle refocusing trains. Proceeding of the International Society of Magnetic Resonance in Medicine 2003;11:206.

[21] Greenman RL, Shirosky JE, Mulkern RV, et al. Double inversion black-blood fast spin-echo imaging of the human heart: a comparison between 1.5T and 3.0T. J Magn Reson Imaging 2003;17:648–55.

[22] Alsop D, Watkins RD, Greenman R, et al. In-vivo mapping of B1 uniformity produced by a whole body 3T RF coil. Proceeding of the International Society of Magnetic Resonance in Medicine 2001;9:1094.

[23] Kangarlu A, Baertlein BA, Lee R, et al. Dielectric resonance phenomena in ultra high field MRI. J Comput Assist Tomogr 1999;23:821–31.

[24] Hussain SM, De Becker J, Hop WCJ, et al. Can a single-shot black-blood T2-weighted spin-echo echo planar imaging sequence with sensitivity encoding replace the respiratory-triggered turbo spin-echo sequence for the liver?—an optimization and a feasibility study. J Magn Reson Imaging 2005;21:219–29.

[25] Nobauer-Huhmann IM, Ba-Ssalamah A, Mlynarik V, et al. Magnetic resonance imaging contrast enhancement of brain tumors at 3 tesla versus 1.5 tesla. Invest Radiol 2002;37: 114–9.

[26] Morakkabati-Spitz N, Schild HH, Kuhl CK, et al. Female pelvis: MR imaging at 3.0 T with sensitivity encoding and flip-angle sweep technique. Radiology 2006;241:538–45.

[27] Van den Bos IC, Hussain SM, Krestin GP, et al. Variable-rate-selective-excitation (VERSE) RF pulses with fat-suppressed T2-weighted fast spin-echo imaging for breath-hold liver imaging at 3.0T. ESMRMB, 23rd Annual Meeting, Warschau, Poland. Proceeding of the European Society of Magnetic Resonance in Medicine and Biology 2006;108.

[28] Van den Bos IC, Hussain SM, Wielopolski PA. Imaging of the liver at 3.0T: optimization of breath-hold, volumetric fat-suppressed fast spin-echo and diffusion-weighted black-blood echo-planar imaging. ISMRM, 14th Scientific Meeting and Exhibition, Seattle (WA). Proceeding of the International Society of Magnetic Resonance in Medicine 2006;447.

MAGNETIC RESONANCE IMAGING CLINICS

Magn Reson Imaging Clin N Am 14 (2007) 545–548

Index

Note: Page numbers of article titles are in **boldface** type.

1064-9689/07/$ – see front matter © 2007 Elsevier Inc. All rights reserved.
mri.theclinics.com

doi:10.1016/S1064-9689(07)00031-1

Moving?

Make sure your subscription moves with you!

To notify us of your new address, find your **Clinics Account Number** (located on your mailing label above your name), and contact customer service at:

E-mail: elspcs@elsevier.com

800-654-2452 (subscribers in the U.S. & Canada)
407-345-4000 (subscribers outside of the U.S. & Canada)

Fax number: 407-363-9661

Elsevier Periodicals Customer Service
6277 Sea Harbor Drive
Orlando, FL 32887-4800

*To ensure uninterrupted delivery of your subscription, please notify us at least 4 weeks in advance of move.

United States Postal Service
Statement of Ownership, Management, and Circulation

1. Publication Title	2. Publication Number	3. Filing Date
Magnetic Resonance Imaging Clinics of North America	0 1 1 - 1 0 0 9	9/15/06

4. Issue Frequency	5. Number of Issues Published Annually	6. Annual Subscription Price
Feb, May, Aug, Nov	4	$205.00

7. Complete Mailing Address of Known Office of Publication (Not printer) (Street, city, county, state, and ZIP+4)

Elsevier Inc.
360 Park Avenue South
New York, NY 10010-1710

Contact Person
Sarah Carmichael

Telephone
(215) 239-3681

8. Complete Mailing Address of Headquarters or General Business Office of Publisher (Not printer)

Elsevier Inc., 360 Park Avenue South, New York, NY 10010-1710

9. Full Names and Complete Mailing Addresses of Publisher, Editor, and Managing Editor (Do not leave blank)

Publisher (Name and complete mailing address)

John Schrefer, Elsevier Inc., 1600 John F. Kennedy Blvd., Suite 1800, Philadelphia, PA 19103-2899

Editor (Name and complete mailing address)

Barton Dudlick, Elsevier Inc., 1600 John F. Kennedy Blvd., Suite 1800, Philadelphia, PA 19103-2899

Managing Editor (Name and complete mailing address)

Catherine Bewick, Elsevier Inc., 1600 John F. Kennedy Blvd., Suite 1800, Philadelphia, PA 19103-2899

10. Owner (Do not leave blank. If the publication is owned by a corporation, give the name and address of the corporation immediately followed by the names and addresses of all stockholders owning or holding 1 percent or more of the total amount of stock. If not owned by a corporation, give the names and addresses of the individual owners. If owned by a partnership or other unincorporated firm, give its name and address as well as those of each individual owner. If the publication is published by a nonprofit organization, give its name and address.)

Full Name	Complete Mailing Address
Wholly owned subsidiary of	4520 East-West Highway
Reed/Elsevier Inc., US Holdings	Bethesda, MD 20814

11. Known Bondholders, Mortgagees, and Other Security Holders Owning or Holding 1 Percent or More of Total Amount of Bonds, Mortgages, or Other Securities. If none, check box ▶ None

Full Name	Complete Mailing Address
N/A	

12. Tax Status (For completion by nonprofit organizations authorized to mail at nonprofit rates) (Check one)
The purpose, function, and nonprofit status of this organization and the exempt status for federal income tax purposes:
☐ Has Not Changed During Preceding 12 Months
☐ Has Changed During Preceding 12 Months (Publisher must submit explanation of change with this statement)

(See Instructions on Reverse)

PS Form 3526, October 1999

---

13. Publication Title	14. Issue Date for Circulation Data Below
Magnetic Resonance Imaging Clinics of North America	May, 2006

15. Extent and Nature of Circulation			Average No. Copies Each Issue During Preceding 12 Months	No. Copies of Single Issue Published Nearest to Filing Date
a.	Total Number of Copies (Net press run)		4,800	4,800
b. Paid and/or Requested Circulation	(1)	Paid/Requested Outside-County Mail Subscriptions Stated on Form 3541. (Include advertiser's proof and exchange copies)	2,902	2,761
	(2)	Paid In-County Subscriptions Stated on Form 3541 (Include advertiser's proof and exchange copies)		
	(3)	Sales Through Dealers and Carriers, Street Vendors, Counter Sales, and Other Non-USPS Paid Distribution	813	793
	(4)	Other Classes Mailed Through the USPS		
c.	Total Paid and/or Requested Circulation (Sum of 15b. (1), (2), (3), and (4))	▶	3,715	3,554
d. Free Distribution by Mail (Samples, complimentary, and other free)	(1)	Outside-County as Stated on Form 3541	129	139
	(2)	In-County as Stated on Form 3541		
	(3)	Other Classes Mailed Through the USPS		
e.	Free Distribution Outside the Mail (Carriers or other means)			
f.	Total Free Distribution (Sum of 15d. and 15e.)	▶	129	139
g.	Total Distribution (Sum of 15c. and 15f.)	▶	3,844	3,693
h.	Copies not Distributed		956	1,107
i.	Total (Sum of 15g. and h.)	▶	4,800	4,800
j.	Percent Paid and/or Requested Circulation (15c. divided by 15g. times 100)		96.64%	96.24%

16. Publication of Statement of Ownership
☒ Publication required. Will be printed in the November 2006 issue of this publication.
☐ Publication not required

17. Signature and Title of Editor, Publisher, Business Manager, or Owner

[signature] Paul Fancier – Executive Director of Subscription Services

Date 9/15/06

I certify that all information furnished on this form is true and complete. I understand that anyone who furnishes false or misleading information on this form or who omits material or information requested on the form may be subject to criminal sanctions (including fines and imprisonment) and/or civil sanctions (including civil penalties).

Instructions to Publishers

1. Complete and file one copy of this form with your postmaster annually on or before October 1. Keep a copy of the completed form for your records.
2. In cases where the stockholder or security holder is a trustee, include in items 10 and 11 the name of the person or corporation for whom the trustee is acting. Also include the names and addresses of individuals who own or hold 1 percent or more of the total amount of bonds, mortgages, or other securities of the publishing corporation. In item 11, if none, check the box. Use blank sheets if more space is required.
3. Be sure to furnish all circulation information called for in item 15. Free circulation must be shown in items 15d, e, and f.
4. Item 15h., Copies not Distributed, must include (1) newsstand copies originally stated on Form 3541, and returned to the publisher, (2) estimated returns from news agents, and (3), copies for office use, leftovers, spoiled, and all other copies not distributed.
5. If the publication had Periodicals authorization as a general or requester publication, this Statement of Ownership, Management, and Circulation must be published; it must be printed in any issue in October or, if the publication is not published during October, the first issue printed after October.
6. In item 16, indicate the date of the issue in which this Statement of Ownership will be published.
7. Item 17 must be signed.
Failure to file or publish a statement of ownership may lead to suspension of Periodicals authorization.

PS Form 3526, October 1999 (Reverse)